江苏省十四五教育科学规划2022年度省重点课题（编号B/2022/01/79）

新医科学术英语读写指南

主 编 钟家宝 朱九扬

副主编 朱春梅 刘慎军

刘 冰 赵 静

U0250417

南京大学出版社

图书在版编目(CIP)数据

新医科学术英语读写指南 / 钟家宝，朱九扬主编.
—南京：南京大学出版社，2024.8
（学科英语系列丛书 / 钟家宝主编）
ISBN 978 - 7 - 305 - 27073 - 4

Ⅰ.①新⋯　Ⅱ.①钟⋯ ②朱⋯　Ⅲ.①医学－英语－
阅读教学－高等学校－教材②医学－英语－写作－高等学
校－教材　Ⅳ.①R

中国国家版本馆 CIP 数据核字(2023)第 100539 号

出版发行　南京大学出版社
社　　址　南京市汉口路 22 号　　　　　邮　　编　210093
丛 书 名　学科英语系列丛书
丛书主编　钟家宝
书　　名　**新医科学术英语读写指南**
　　　　　XINYIKE XUESHU YINGYU DUXIE ZHINAN
主　　编　钟家宝　朱九扬
责任编辑　张淑文　　　　　　　　编辑热线　(025)83592401
照　　排　南京开卷文化传媒有限公司
印　　刷　南京百花彩色印刷广告制作有限责任公司
开　　本　787 mm×1092 mm　1/16 开　印张 14.5　字数 470 千
版　　次　2024 年 8 月第 1 版　2024 年 8 月第 1 次印刷
ISBN 978 - 7 - 305 - 27073 - 4
定　　价　50.00 元

网　　址：http://www.njupco.com
官方微博：http://weibo.com/njupco
微信服务号：njuyuexue
销售咨询热线：(025)83594756

Contents

Unit 1
Reading and Writing an Abstract

The abstract is an important section of a research paper and often encourages the reader to continue reading the article. Writing a working abstract not only provides the writer with a framework for the article, but also avoids reworking drearily. Researchers publishing in medical research journals turn to a basic structure of research article. A structured abstract is generally required: Background, Method, Results, Discussion, and Conclusions.

Highlight

In this unit, you will

- Learn vocabulary to help you express precision medicine terms and write a working abstract
- Learn the conventions of sentence writing and paragraph structure
- Identify reliable sources of academic information
- Recognize and write about key terms of precision medicine
- Write a definition for a precision medicine term
- Write a working abstract for a research paper on precision medicine
- Build a model for a working abstract

Gearing up

Work in a small group, and discuss the following questions. When you have finished, share your answers with the class.

1. How would you define an abstract?
2. How would you define a structured abstract?
3. What type of information should be in an abstract, and in what order?
4. What are the differences between traditional abstracts and structured abstracts?
5. Do you believe writing abstract needs a model? Why?

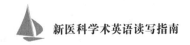

Section 1　Reading

Task 1　Activating background knowledge

Task 1A　Work in pairs and discuss the following questions.

1. What is academic reading?
2. What difficulties do you have when reading academic texts?

Look at Table 1.1 and tick your items，then share your answers with your classmates.

Table 1.1　Questionnaire for difficulties in academic reading

Difficulties in academic reading	Very easy	Easy	Difficult	Very difficult
Identifying main ideas				
Identifying supporting sentences				
Understanding terms				
Understanding the organization of a genre				
Recreating the meaning of a discourse				
Working out the meaning of an unfamiliar word				

Task 1B　To help you to read academic genre effectively，here are some steps in Table 1.2 that you are required to tick.

Table 1.2　Questionnaire for steps in academic reading

Steps	Yes	No
Pre-reading provides an overview of the content and tone of what is read		
Skimming is to find the topic sentence，key words and phrases		
Academic readers negotiate the meaning with the author by applying their prior knowledge to it		
Use your knowledge of the genre structure to predict the organization of the text		

Task 2　Understanding the facts and details

Reading 1　Text theme：Precision medicine

Task 2A　Read the text，and fill in each blank with a proper form of the word in the bracket.

Improving Public Cancer Care by Implementing Precision Medicine
Aslaud Helland, et al

Background: Matching treatment based on tumour molecular characteristics has revolutionized the treatment of some cancers and has given hope to many patients. Although personalized cancer care is an old concept, renewed attention has arisen due to recent advancements in cancer diagnostics including access to high throughput sequencing of tumour tissue. _____ (targeting) therapies interfering with cancer specific pathways have been developed and approved for subgroups of patients. These drugs might just as well be efficient in other diagnostic subgroups, not investigated in pharma led clinical studies, but their potential use on new _____ (indicators) is never explored due to limited number of patients.

Methods: In this national, investigator initiated, prospected, open labels, non randomized combined basket and umbrella trial, patients are enrolled in multiple _____ (paralleled) cohorts. Each cohort is defined by the patient's tumour type, molecular profile of the tumour, and study drug. Treatment outcome in each cohort is monitored by using a Simon two stage like 'admissible' monitoring plan to identity evidence of clinical activity. All drugs available in IMPRESS Norway have regulatory approval and are funded by pharmaceutical companies. Molecular diagnostics are _____ (funder) by the public health care system.

Discussion: _____ (precise) oncology means to stratify treatment based on specific patient characteristics and the molecular profile of the tumor. Use of targeted drugs is currently restricted to specific biomarker defined subgroups of patients according to their market authorization. However, other cancer patients might also benefit of treatment with these drugs if the same biomarker is present. The emerging technologies in molecular diagnostics are now being _____ (implementing) in Norway and it is publicly reimbursed, thus more cancer patients will have a more comprehensive genomic profiling of their tumour. Patients with actionable genomic alternation in their tumour may have the possibility to try precision cancer drugs through IMPRESS Norway, if standard treatment is no longer an option, and the drugs are available in the study. This might benefit some patients. In addition, it is a good example of a public-private collaboration to establish a national infrastructure for precision oncology.

From J Transl Med., 2022, 20(1):225

Task 2B Read the text carefully. Decide whether these statements are TRUE (T) or FALSE (F).

1. Targeted therapies interfering with cancer specific pathways have been

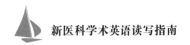

developed and approved for subgroups of patients. （　）
2. Molecular diagnostics is funded by pharmaceutical companies. （　）
3. Precision oncology means to stratify treatment based on specific patient characteristics and the molecular profile of the tumor. （　）
4. The study is a good example of a public-private collaboration to establish a pharmaceutical company's infrastructure for precision oncology. （　）

Task 3　Academic literacy skills: Read for specific information

Task 3A　Search and identify reliable sources of information

Using reliable sources in the academic environment is of vital importance. Discuss the following sources of academic information with your classmates, and check your skills of identifying reliable scientific sources. Tick those to which you may say yes.

Sources	Verified		Biased		Data-based		Peer-reviewed		Reliable	
	full	part	full	part	full	part	full	part	full	part
Textbooks										
Dictionaries										
Journal articles										
Newspapers and magazines										
Online academic blogs										
Online data sources										
Online search tools										

Task 3B　Moves in structured abstracts

The abstracts generally follow a five-move pattern depending on the type of abstract involved and the communicative function that it serves: relation to other research, purpose, methodology, results and discussion of the research (Cross & Oppenheim, 2006). A typical structured abstract is written by using five sub-headings—"background", "aim/purpose", "method", "results" and "conclusions" (Hartley, 2008). Most well-structured medical English abstracts follow a four or five-move pattern. The basic core structure of four-moves is "purpose/aim", "patients/methods", "results" and "conclusion", "statement of the problem/background" and "recommendations" are optional moves (Salager-Meyer, 1990).

Task 4　Understanding the text moves

Reading 2　Text theme: Precision medicine in oncology
Task 4A　Read the text and fill in each blank with a proper form of the word in

the bracket.

Comprehensive Genome Profiling in Patients With Metastatic Non-Small Cell Lung Cancer: The Precision Medicine Phase Ⅱ Randomized SAFIR02-Lung Trial

Fabrice Barles et al

Purpose: Targeted therapies (TT) and immune checkpoint blockers (ICB) have revolutionized the approach to non-small cell lung cancer (NSCLC) treatment in the era of precision medicine. Their _____ (impacting) as switch maintenance therapy based on molecular characterization is unknown.

Patients and Methods: SAFIR02-Lung was an open-label, randomized, phase II trial, involving 33 centers in France. We investigated eight TT (substudy-1) and one ICB (substudy-2), compared with standard-of-care as a _____ (maintain) strategy in patients with advanced EGFR, ALK wild-type (wt) NSCLC without progression after first-line chemotherapy, based on high-throughput genome analysis. The primary outcome was progression-free survival (PFS).

Results: Among the 175 patients randomized in substudy-1, 116 received TT (selumetinib, vistusertib, capivasertib, AZD4547, AZD8931, vandetanib, olaparib, savolitinib) and 59 standard-of care. Median PFS was 2.7 months [95% confidence intervals (CI), 1.6—2.9] with TT versus 2.7 months (1.6—4.1) with standard-of-care (HR, 0.97; 95% CI, 0.7—1.36; P ¼ 0.87). There were no significant differences in PFS within any molecular subgroup. In substudy-2, 183 patients were randomized, 121 received durvalumab and 62 standard-of-care. Median PFS was 3.0 months (2.3—4.4) with durvalumab versus 3.0 months (2.0—5.1) with standard-of-care (HR, 0.86; 95% CI, 0.62—1.20; P = 0.38). Preplanned subgroup analysis showed an _____ (enhance) benefit with durvalumab in patients with PD-L1 tumor proportion score (TPS) $\geqslant$1%, (n = 29; HR, 0.29; 95% CI, 0.11—0.75) as compared with PD-L1<1% (n = 31; HR, 0.71; 95% CI, 0.31—1.60; $P_{interaction}$ = 0.036).

Conclusions: Molecular profiling can feasibly be implemented to guide treatment choice for the maintainance strategy in EGFR/ALK wt NSCLC; in this study it did not lead to substantial treatment benefits beyond durvalumab for PD-L1 $\geqslant$ 1 patients.

From Clin Cancer Res., 2022, 28(18)

Task 4B   Read the text carefully and decide what the moves are.
1. What are the contents of the clinical experiment? Which section tells you?
2. What is the background of the clinical research?
3. What are the limitations of the clinical research?

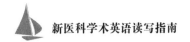

Task 5　Building your vocabulary

Work with your partner，match each key word and phrase from Reading 1 or Reading 2 to its definition.

Word/phrase	Definition
1. potential	**a.** the act of working with another person or group of people to create or produce sth
2. implemented	**b.** the inherent capacity for coming into being
3. precision	**c.** forced or compelled or put in force
4. enhanced	**d.** the quality of being reproducible in amount or performance
5. maintenance	**e.** increased or intensified in value or beauty or quality
6. survival	**f.** activity involved in maintaining something in good working order
7. proportion	**g.** a natural process resulting in the evolution of organisms best adapted to the environment
8. involve	**h.** the quotient obtained when the magnitude of a part is divided by the magnitude of the whole.
9. impact	**i.** connect closely and often incriminatingly
10. investigate	**j.** the striking of one body against another
11. label	**k.** conduct an inquiry or investigation of
12. therapy	**l.** attach a tag or label to
13. randomize	**m.** heat therapy gave the best relief
14. tumor	**n.** to use a method in an experiment，a piece of research，etc. that gives every item an equal chance of being considered；to put things in a random order
15. treatment	**o.** an abnormal new mass of tissue that serves no purpose
16. diagnostics	**p.** something that is done to cure an illness or injury，or to make sb look and feel good
17. precision oncology	**q.** the art or practice of diagnosis，esp of diseases
18. subgroup	**r.** stratify treatment based on specific patient characteristics and the molecular profile of the tumor.
19. collaboration	**s.** a smaller group made up of members of a larger group

Section 2   Writing

Task 6   Warm-up writing assignment

Task 6A   Verb tense, modality and phraseology in medical abstracts.

1. Verb tense

The tense distribution in medical abstracts varies with the abstract rhetorical moves. The tenses used in decreasing order of frequency are usually the past, present, and present perfect, and usually in active voice. In the purpose move, the tense is basically past or present. In order to express the role of an obligatory constraint, the past tense and passive voice are used in the materials/methods move of medical abstracts. The present tense is frequently used in the conclusions, implications and recommendation sections of a research paper. The present perfect is recognized as the tense markers of the statement of the problem and is essentially used to introduce a topic of the text.

The modals of high frequency in scientific writing are May, Can, Should, which can establish the discoursal function of signalling the more tentative, suggestive conclusion, data synthesis, and recommendation moves (Salager-Meyer, 1992).

2. Modality

Search for distribution frequency of verbs and modals from more than 10 medical abstracts of research papers, and fill in the following table for distribution tenses and modals of medical English abstracts.

Tense, voice or modal	Move					
	Statement of the problem/ background	Purpose	Materials/ methods/ patients	Results/ findings	Conclusions	Recommendations
Present						
Active						
Passive						
Past						
Active						
Passive						
Pr Pf						
Active						

Continued

Tense, voice or modal	Move					
	Statement of the problem/ background	Purpose	Materials/ methods/ patients	Results/ findings	Conclusions	Recommendations
Passive						
Future						
Active						
Passive						
Ps Pf						
Active						
Passive						
May						
Can						
Should						
Must						
Could						
Might						

Note：Pr Pf = present perfect，Ps Pf = past perfect，Active = active voice，Passive = passive voice

3. Phraseology in medical abstracts

Verb tense is especially important in an abstract for strict word limit. Phrases associated with all these moves are listed below.

（1）The tense for describing the importance of the topic and reference to the literature is the present and the present perfect tense，the following are some examples.

> During brain development...**plays** an essential **role** for establishing...
>
> ...increasingly **recognize**(s) a **need** for assistance from...
>
> ...has been **recognised** as the...
>
> There has been **recent renewed interest** in studying human early...
>
> A **renewed interest** in...research has led to the discovery of several novel human...
>
> **Recent** studies have shown a **renewed interest** in...
>
> **Changes** in the short-term dynamics of... over development have been **observed** throughout...
>
> Although **much research** has been done **investigating** the roles of...

Previous research has found positive **associations** between... and aerobic fitness...

Previous studies have **indicated** an **association** between...

Prior **studies** have **documented** that access to testing has not been equitable...

Previous **studies** demonstrate poor delirium documentation rates in...

In this article, we investigate the **importance** of phase for...

It is suggested that **attempts** to offer such a description are...

Some **attempt** has been **made** to discover if the average person is...

A **growing body** of literature **suggests** that...plays a critical role in...

The **evidence suggests** that...consumption can decrease...

Although the...has not yet been fully elucidated, a **growing body** of **evidence suggests** that...

...is rapidly **becoming** a popular **trend**...

There is an increasing **trend** of performing...

(2) The present simple tense is generally used for the statement/identification of a knowledge gap/problem, the following are some examples.

The **problem** is likely to be most acute in cases of deep...

In this paper, we consider the **problem** of fair statistical inference involving...

It is shown that the **problem** is a special case of a more general class...

The main **problem**, however, is...

...properties are not well **understood yet**.

...yet we remain **largely ignorant** of the mechanisms by which successful vaccines...

...health professionals are **largely ignorant** of the condition...

The etiology of this condition is **still poorly understood**, although...

However, this assumption is **not valid** when...

(3) When you are referring to the purpose/aim of the current study, you may use the present simple tense or the past tense, the following are some examples.

This **study aims** to review the use of smart phones and social media in the context of...

The **aim** of this **study** was to evaluate the…of the nasopalatine canal in…

This **study examines** the practical implications of…in the context of…

The current **study set out to examine** motor intentions…plant behavior…

We **set out to confirm** this and **whether** any…diagnosis was responsible for…

The **principal objective** of this **project** was to **investigate** the effects of…

Thus, this **research aimed** to **explore** the underlying association between…

The studies aimed at **exploring** the link between…and…are scarce.

The **present study aimed** to characterize the **relationship** using contrast…

This **paper presents** a **new**… method with evaporative light scattering detection…

This **paper aims** at providing…evaluation **approaches**…

(4) When you are referring to your materials/methodology/process, it is common to use the past simple tense, the following are some examples.

Changes to their daily lives were **examined** through the lens of…

A simulated **sample** was successfully **prepared** and possessed…

Phase separation upon heating was **investigated** in salt solutions of…

A variety of textual, ethnographic, and historical **materials** are **examined**…

The questionnaire was designed to **provide quantitative**…of clinical pain…

Clinical data were **collected** both…using parent **questionnaires** and medical records…

…the data were **collected** via an online **questionnaire**.

A quasi-experimental **design** with…**control groups** was used in this **study**.

(5) It is also likely to use the present simple tense to describe your materials/methodology, especially when you are illustrating calculations or equations which can be found in the paper itself, the following are some examples.

Numerical examples are **analysed** in detail…

Peers chosen using the preferred models are **compared** with…

These metaheuristic algorithms are **created** by modifying their logical structure via…

The exact specifications…outlined for making **comparisons** are explicated from quotes…

The stages of the **method** are **illustrated** using examples from...

The application of the **methods** is **illustrated** with data from..

The **case studies** are organised into **four** categories related to...

The current **study provides** a **novel approach** to **quantify**...risk factors of...

This **study** introduces a generalized **approach** for **quantifying** parameter uncertainty...

We also design a holdout **approach** to **identify**... significantly associated with...

Our **approach identifies** expression traits that have...associations...

...but there is no **quantitative data** characterizing and benchmarking...

It represents an...approach，combining **qualitative and quantitative** research approaches...

（6）Results/findings can be expressed in either the present simple tense，or the present past tense，the following are some examples.

We **find** that this inescapable property of... curvature has important consequences for...

We **find** that a large share of the...respond by substituting Medicaid for...

The evaluation results **showed** that the performance of the...**model** was poor as it **consistently underpredicted**...

We **found** that the majority of **model** outputs **underpredicted** the measured...

Several **examples** illustrate how such materials...

We selected two **examples** among...as a good illustration of how catalysis makes...

The earliest and most **marked increases** in young women occurred in...

Bleeding was **observed** only in the groups of clinical comparison 1 and 2...

The majority of respondents **consistently** chose... variance plan，**consistent** with...utility theory.

Results revealed that the **consistency** of the product varied with...

ANOVAs indicated that only fatigue-inertia and... were significantly **affected** by...

Analysis of the data showed that...administration did not **affect** mood，but significant...

...challenge is to identify alterations in...associated with distinct **profiles** of negative **affect**...

All imaging results should be **correlated** with the patient's **signs** and **symptoms**...

Results of this blood flow are mixed with the beneficial effects of removing...

The **results** revealed that a variable pressure boundary causes a...

...successfully assigned irreversible, deterministic **identifiers** to survey...

Studies were **identified** through a search of the electronic databases...

Only half of the **respondents reported** that all colleagues at their site followed...

Respondents used frequency scales to **report** how often they access both...and...

(7) Even if the subject sentence is in the past simple tense (The result showed/It was showed etc.), we can decide to use present simple tense to express the finding/result itself or the implication of the result if we believe it is to be considered as a fact or truth.

Clinical trials **showed that** cancer anorexia **should be** considered as... encompassing different...

...we **found** that...signaling pathways **might be** involved in testicular injury due to...

The experiments **demonstrated** there **are** two matrices...

It **was found** that proteins **are** produced from...

This finding **suggested** that there **is** a direct relationship between...

(8) Achievement/applications/discussion/conclusion/can be expressed in the present perfect tense, the past simple tense or the present simple tense.

In conclusion, the ANN **was proven to** be an innovative methodology for interpreting...

The findings of our study **provide**... support for the acceptability and feasibility of adopting...

Our results **revealed** substantial recommendations for refining navigation, layout and...

Identifying the dimensions with...scores **allowed** the institution's managers to concentrate...

The analysis **shows** that the tendency to remove...practices from moral evaluation by...

Overall，this... counseling **application can provide** a valuable and... communication...

To summarize，when you describe a patient as...it **implies** the...

This **implies** that... monitoring can provide sufficient information for understanding...

There is **clear evidence** that refrigerated platelets are **cleared** by...

The implication of...in the pathogenesis of human asthma **seems** to be more and more likely...

Many advances **have been made to implicate**...in clinical trials...

We **highlight** the importance of...and thorough investigations especially in children...

The present study **highlights** how implantation mismatches may affect the...

As a result of these investigations，suggestions **were identified** for future research...

It **was concluded** that this initial survey **had revealed** important information about the...

Demonstrations **are** automatically **decomposed** into...sub-behaviors which allows the...

This chip **provides** a **powerful tool** for immunogenetics gene mapping...

Task 6B　Sentence structure and paragraph structure

1. Sentence structure

（1）A minimal/simple sentence

The basic principle in written English illustrates that sentence units occur in integration，and in relationship to other sentence elements，most sentences contain a Subject→Verb structure. The subject always precedes the verb，except in questions where the order is reversed.

Subject	Verb Predicate	
Oslo University Hospital	is	the sponsor of the study
Patients	will be treated	at their local hospital...
We	analyzed	mutation spectra in 16 patients...

The subject is the topic or theme of the sentence，which may be one word，but the contexts in which sentence elements occur determine the variation among them.

Subjects can be filled by all kinds of words or phrases, such as proper and common nouns, countable and uncountable nouns, abstract and concrete nouns, compound noun phrases and sets of parallel.

The predicate is one part of a sentence, which can indicate an action, a state, or simply serve to link the subject to other information, and it may also consist of a predicate verb with or without any complementation. Various other sentence elements may be placed before or after the Subject→Verb structure.

Subject	Verb Predicate	
Chimeric antigen receptor T-cell therapies targeting CD19	have demonstrated	manageable safety profiles and high efficacy in the treatment of relapsed/ refractory...
All 40 treated patients	met	the eligibility criteria for having high-risk disease
This	is	the first report of the feasibility of comprehensive molecular...
Complete response rates and ORRs among key subgroups generally	aligned with	the overall patient population...

(2) Complex sentences

Many sentences contain more than one Subject → Verb structure, which are organized by a hierarchy based on their importance for a sentence to be grammatical, but one of these parts will convey the main meaning and will make sense by itself.

Adverb/prepositional phrase	Subject noun phrase	Predicate verb phrase	Object noun phrase
Beyond identification of somatic actionable alterations	broad genomic profiling	possesses	the advantage to uncover precious information...
At present,	existing precision oncology trials	predominantly address	patients in a metastatic incurable situation...
In conclusion,	our findings from the primary analysis of ZUMA12	provide	evidence that axi-cel is safe and highly effective...

(3) Compound sentences

Some sentences may have two parts that contain one Subject → Verb structure themself, and both of them convey meaning that can make sense by itself. They may be joined by words like and, or, but, so, or a semi-colon.

Subject	Verb Predicate	Object noun phrase
The comparator	will contain	an aggregated group of patients...
Genetic ancestry data	may facilitate	more nuanced and equitable use of precision medicine...
This group	will gradually be refined to match	the treated patients
Patients from racial and ethnic minority groups	remain underrepresented	in much of this work

2. Paragraph structure

A paragraph is a series of related sentences that develop the main idea clearly. Most paragraphs in an academic essay contain a topic sentence and supporting sentences, and some paragraphs also have a transitional sentence or/and a concluding sentence (Oshima & Hogue, 2007).

(1) Read the following paragraph carefully, and then analyze its structure.

① Congenital Disorders of Glycosylation (CDG) are a rapidly growing family of rare monogenic metabolic conditions. ② A hundred and fifty-seven genes have been linked to CDG, resulting in high intra and inter-disease clinical heterogeneity. ③ PMM2-CDG (MIM: 212065) was the first reported N-glycosylation defect and remains the most common CDG worldwide. ④ CDG biological complexies, associated research funding limitations, disease expert and patient dispersion and scarcity hinder robust data collection. ⑤ These challenges prevent full elucidation of CDG clinical picture(s) and of their natural history with immunological involvement remaining one of the least well-characterized manifestations (Francisco et al. (2022). The road to successful people-centric research in rare diseases: the web-based case study of the Immunology and Congenital Disorders of Glycosylation questionnaire (ImmunoCDGQ). *From Orphanet Journal of Rare Diseases, 17(134): 1-18.*

The topic sentence states the main idea of the paragraph. It consists of the topic and the controlling idea which is made about the topic, and is the most important sentence in a paragraph. It briefly indicates what the paragraph is going to discuss.

　　　　Topic　　　　　　　　　　　　　　　　　**Controlling idea**

Congenital Disorders of Glycosylation (CDG) are a rapidly growing family of rare monogenic metabolic conditions.

Supporting sentences develop the topic sentence by giving specific details about the topic. That is, they explain or prove the topic sentence by giving reasons, examples, facts, statistics, and quotations. The following supporting sentences explain the topic sentence about Congenital Disorders of Glycosylation.

A hundred and fifty-seven genes have been linked to CDG, resulting in high intra and inter-disease clinical heterogeneity.

PMM2-CDG（MIM: 212065）was the first reported N-glycosylation defect and remains the most common CDG worldwide.

CDG biological complexities, associated research funding limitations, disease expert and patient dispersion and scarcity hinder robust data collection.

The concluding sentence signals the end of the paragraph and leaves the reader with important points to remember. It tells the reader that the paragraph is finished.

E.g. These challenges prevent full elucidation of CDG clinical picture(s) and of their natural history with immunological involvement remaining one of the least well-characterized manifestations

(2) Identify the parts of a topic sentence. Underline the topic and the controlling idea in each of the sentences below, and discuss the ways of recognizing the topic sentence with your classmates.

① Assigned race is a social construct, but racism has biological consequences.

② Investigators should be cognizant of the ways that our current research practices perpetuate inequities in cancer care.

③ The expansion of both e-research tools and patient-centricity approaches have underlined the need to effectively educate patients in order to provide them with a skill set that supports their active and meaningful involvement in research.

④ Each tumour type/molecular variant/drug will define a specific cohort, and each cohort constitutes a Simon two stage trial model to identify cohorts with evidence of clinical activity.

⑤ Patients with advanced malignancies are eligible after disease progression on standard treatment.

⑥ The advent of precision medicine has dramatically revolutionized the landscape of cancer treatment.

⑦ Several studies have confirmed the feasibility of implementing NGS in therapeutic decision-making in patients with advanced cancer.

⑧ Eligible patients received four cycles of platinum-based chemotherapy according to local standard practice.

(3) Write topic sentences for the following paragraphs.

Topic sentence: _____.

      Language barriers, lack of insurance coverage, geographic and financial barriers, as well as system level barriers such as limited time by oncologists are barriers to receipt of evidence-based cancer care, including precision medicine, among these populations. Patient knowledge of precision medicine is associated with increased participation in precision medicine research and receipt of precision cancer care such as targeted therapy. However, precision medicine is a difficult concept to discuss and comprehend overall and minority populations report less comprehension than White populations likely due to lower rates of clinician-directed discussions regarding these topics among these populations. Increased knowledge about precision medicine among minorities, therefore, is a critical step in closing the gap in cancer mortality rates, especially as precision medicine continues to advance.

Topic sentence: _____.

      In our previous work, CHWs integrated into cancer care delivery have also effectively increased advance care planning, reduced symptom burden and reduced acute care use among patients with advanced stages of cancer. However, less is known about the effectiveness of CHWs in educating patients about precision medicine (basic concepts of genetic testing, tumor testing and targeted therapies), and no randomized trial, to our knowledge, has evaluated the effectiveness of such an approach among low-income and racial and ethnic minority adults.

Topic sentence: _____.

      Despite significantly higher cure rates due to improved earlier diagnosis and interdisciplinary standard-of-care (SoC) treatment, BC remains the leading cause of tumor-related deaths in women worldwide, with reports estimating 685 000 deaths annually. SoC of high-risk early BC includes cytotoxic chemotherapy, which is preferentially administered as a preoperative neoadjuvant chemotherapy (NACT). Given the close correlation between residual cancer burden after NACT and outcome, NACT outperforms adjuvant therapy regimens due to the prospect for early in vivo efficacy assessment of the administered therapy. This strategy facilitates the identification of high-risk patients at the timepoint of surgery, who have a poor prognosis, allowing to dynamically adapt and escalate therapeutic interventions before overt metastatic disease develops.

(4) Write supporting sentences to explain or prove the following topic sentences with examples, statistics or quotations.

① Technological advances, namely those based on the internet have opened promising avenues not only for clinical care but also for biomedical research, particularly in the field of rare diseases (RDs). Web-based platforms have several advantages and address various gaps, namely: _____ [1]. Several international initiatives have been exploring these e-health and e-research pathways. _____ [2]. Additionally, there is the Share4Rare web-platform that congregates multi-RD research projects and the Rare Barometer e-survey program. _____ [3].

② Another advantage of umbrella trials for screening is that it is possible to cycle quickly through ineffective treatments. _____ [1]. For example, _____ [2]. The GBM AGILE (Glioblastoma adaptive, global, innovative learning environment) trial (NCT03970447) implements a seamless phase Ⅱ/Ⅲ response-adaptive platform design. In this trial, treatment arms that show success in the first part of the trial can graduate to the next stage for confirmation through the interim analysis. Additionally, the adaptive adjustment of randomization probabilities at the interims allows the trial resource to be focused on the sub-studies with more promising results, thus accelerates the testing of new precision oncology treatments. Gajewski et al. further _____ [3].

③ Precision oncology trials offer treatment options by application of drugs targeting molecular alterations detected in tumor cells via genomic and/or transcriptomic profiling approaches. For example, _____ [1]. So far, however, this approach has been mainly confined to the palliative setting. _____ [2], with the prospect to apply and validate targeted molecular therapies also within post-neoadjuvant settings.

(5) Write concluding sentences to finish the paragraph or highlight the important ideas by summarizing the main ideas or repeating the topic of the paragraph.

① Precision medicine remains relatively novel within gynecologic oncology, reflected by the numerous, recently opened precision oncology trials in gynecologic cancers. These ongoing trials offer a meaningful opportunity for investigators to directly address the ways inequitable enrollment patterns characterized in our study perpetuate gynecologic cancer disparities. Improving trial representation across racial and ethnic groups may be accomplished through a variety of interventions; reliance on patient self-report, diverse research teams—especially at the investigator level, hospital-level interventions such as physician implicit bias and communication training, patient and community participation in trial design and recruitment strategies, and active collaboration between trial sites to adjust recruitment goals based on regional demographics._____

_____ .

② Efforts to expand treatment options for gynecologic cancers may be limited by available funding opportunities. Only 30.9% of trials in our study received National Institutes of Health funding compared with approximately 60.0% of U.S.-based precision oncology trials in prostate cancer. Prostate cancer and gynecologic cancers each cause 30,000 deaths annually. However, the estimated 5-year survival of prostate cancer is 96.8% compared with 81.3%, 66.7%, and 49.7% for uterine, cervical and ovarian cancers, respectively. Lack of _____

_____ .

③ This is the first report of the feasibility of comprehensive molecular profiling and its clinical applicability within the molecular precision registry trial COGNITION for patients with early BC with NACT indication. We carried out WGS/WES and RNA sequencing to identify molecular targets for individualized post-neoadjuvant treatment of patients who are still at high risk for relapse following SoC NACT and surgery. Thus COGNITON is _____

_____ .

3. Paragraph organization

The organization of the paragraph is to develop your ideas in some kinds of order, such as chronological order, logical division of ideas, and comparison/contrast.

(1) Discuss the steps of chronological order, logical division of ideas, and comparison/contrast with your classmates.

(2) Read the following paragraphs and rearrange the sentences in logical order.

[1] ① Postoperative infectious complications are a major source of morbidity, resulting in an increased hospital length of stay (LOS), a delay in chemotherapy, and a worse cancer prognosis. ② The underlying cause for postoperative infections is the profound immune suppression in response to surgery-induced changes, such as nutritional deficiencies and inflammatory signals. ③ Surgical resection is the primary curative treatment for most solid malignancies, including colorectal cancer (CRC).

[2] ① Patients with both impaired renal function and borderline functional

19

status experienced even higher rates of severe acute toxicity, questioning the role of platinum-based regimens in this context. ② Treatment options for cisplatin-ineligible patients are limited. ③ The EORTC 30986 trial compared the combination of gemcitabine plus carboplatin（GCa）versus methotrexate, carboplatin, plus vinblastine （M-CAVI）and demonstrated severe acute toxicity in 9.3% of patients receiving GCa and 21.2% of patients receiving M-CAVI.

[3] ① There are approximately six million people with Alzheimer's disease in the United States, and at least one study estimates that it has become the third leading cause of death. ② Neurodegenerative diseases such as Alzheimer's disease, frontotemporal dementia, and amyotrophic lateral sclerosis are without effective therapeutics. ③ Unfortunately, therapeutic approaches to date have not led to sustainable improvements, and the best results from recent clinical trials have been to slow cognitive decline rather than improve cognition or halt decline.

Task 6C Write definitions

1. Writing definitions are generally needed in different academic situations. Here are some suggestions that you offer a definition for a term or concept. Tick your answer in the table below and discuss with your classmates.

Situations	YES	NO
To clarify a word or phrase in the title		
To make a term familiar to your readers		
To display your understanding of a course paper or examination		
To explain a technical word or phrase		
To illustrate a word or phrase with some ambiguious meanings		
To shed light on the meaning of the original term		

2. The definitions in the following table have been mixed up. Discuss with your partner and rewrite them.

Concept	Category	Detail	Use
(1) Breast cancer	is a systemic endotheliosis	in women, with 2.3 million newly diagnosed cases	worldwide per year
(2) Migraine	is the most common cancer	worldwide and a major cause of disability	with a substantial social burden

Continued

Concept	Category	Detail	Use
(3) Nitric oxide	is one of the most common diseases	processing noxious impulses and sensitizing	perivascular sensory nerves
(4) Endometriosis	is a non-adrenergic, non-cholinergic neurotransmitter	caused by the growth of the endometrium	from its normal position
(5) Alzheimer's disease	is a disease	now affecting 6.5 million Americans age 65 and older	and projected to double to 13.8 million by 2060
(6) Atypical hemolytic-uremic syndrome	is a devastating neurodegenerative disease	that is characterized by severe microangiopathy and renal failure	leading to uncontrolled activation of the alternative complement pathway
(7) Endometrial carcinoma	are a heterogeneous and complex group of neoplasms	in women, with 320,000 new cases annually,	or 4.8% of cancers in women
(8) Pain during labour	is globally the sixth most common cancer	that many women will experience	during their lives
(9) Posttranslational arginylation	is the most intense pain	catalyzed by the enzyme arginyl-tRNA-transferase, in which amino acid arginine is transferred from tRNA to proteins	in a ribosome-independent manner.
(10) Soft-tissue sarcomas	is a process	of mesenchymal origin,	accounting for only 1% of all cancers

3. Complete the definitions by inserting an appropriate category words.

   (1) Acute myeloid leukemia (AML) is not a single entity but a multitude of _____ that differ with regard to pretreatment genetic features including cytogenetics and gene mutation.

   (2) Multiple sclerosis (MS) is the most common autoimmune _____ of the central nervous system.

   (3) Prostatitis is a prostate _____ characterized by prostate inflammation, pain and a variety of urinary symptoms such as urinary frequency, urgency, dribbling and the need to urinate often at night

   (4) Theoretically, precision exercise is a _____ that could improve the development of basic motor skills, as well as musculoskeletal development and the ability to achieve energy balance and weight control to counteract the acute and long-term effect of treatment and its burdening aftermath.

   (5) Precision exercise is the new _____ in clinical exercise physiology helping to induce oxidative metabolism (i.e. the main system of energy supply within

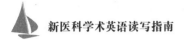

cells) and boost the adaptive response of bones in vulnerable patients.

(6) Depressive syndromes are common in older adults and represent a major public _____ concern.

(7) Cesarean scar pregnancy is a _____ that describes the implantation of a gestational sac at the site of a previous cesarean delivery scar and was first described by Larsen and Solomon in 1978.

(8) Prostate cancer is a major health _____ worldwide and is the second most common cancer in men.

(9) Motor vehicle crashes are the second most common form of traumatic _____ among individuals aged 65 years and older and result in an estimated 250,000 US emergency department visits by older adults each year.

(10) Dry eye is a multifactorial _____ of the tears and ocular surface.

(11) Schizophrenia is a brain _____ characterized by, on average, a reduction in general cognitive abilities of 1 SD below the population mean.

(12) Interpersonal violence is a major _____ of mortality, morbidity and economic cost to society.

4. Complete the following definitions.

(1) Parkinson's disease (PD) is characterized _____ in the substantia nigra pars compacta with resultant depletion of striatal dopamine _____.

(2) Prostate cancer is one of the most frequently _____ and can be an indolent _____.

(3) Synovial sarcoma is _____ of soft tissue that usually arises in the lower extremities near the large _____ of young adults.

(4) Functional disorders are _____ in which there is no obvious _____ or anatomical change in an organ, and there is a presumed _____ of an organ or system.

(5) Knee osteoarthritis is a prevalent _____ in adults throughout the world, resulting in _____, disability, reduced quality of life, and substantial healthcare costs.

(6) Glaucoma is an _____ characterized by progressive degeneration of retinal ganglion cells, leading to _____ to the optic nerve and loss of _____.

(7) Bisphosphonates are _____ that have been widely used in the last years because of their ability to inhibit _____.

(8) Microparticles are a heterogeneous population of _____, with a diameter of 100—1000 nm, released from _____ of various cell types, such as platelets, erythrocytes, granulocytes, monocytes, _____ and endothelial cells.

(9) Low back pain is a highly prevalent and disabling _____ that represents

the major cause of years _____ in both developed and developing countries.

(10) Adductor spasmodic dysphonia is a neurologically based _____ of the laryngeal musculature resulting in a _____, strangled voice quality primarily during speech tasks.

(11) Posterior ankle pain is a cause of _____ pain and disability.

(12) Multiple myeloma is a malignant _____ of the mature B-cell lymphocytes originating in the _____ marrow and may involving the entire _____.

5. Write extensive definitions for the following terms.

(1) Anti-Mullerian hormone is a _____ glycoprotein belonging to _____ _____ superfamily.

(2) Bipolar disorder is a _____ disorder characterized by _____, hypomania and depression, and is often accompanied by _____.

(3) Acute kidney injury is a _____ of critical illness with a large effect on _____.

(4) Traumatic brain injuries (TBI) are a major _____ problem.

(5) Parkinson's disease is a _____ disorder that is caused by selective _____ in the substantia nigra.

(6) Dysregulated metabolism is a cancer _____ and presents opportunities for _____.

(7) Expiratory central airway collapse is defined by _____ collapse during _____, resulting from _____ of the posterior membranous wall.

(8) Autism is a _____ syndrome of the central nervous system, which is _____ by _____ in language and reciprocal social interactions, and a restricted repertoire of _____.

(9) Glucose-6-phosphate dehydrogenase is a key enzyme that _____ the first reaction in the _____.

(10) The human mitochondrial genome is a small (16.5 kb) _____ molecule that is present in _____.

Task 7   Writing task: Build a model

Task 7A Move structures and vocabulary in medical abstracts

1. Move structures

A working abstract will provide a framework for the rest of the article. It is easier to write a working abstract if you know moves of the phrase "structured abstracts" in medical research journals. Structured abstracts include three moves—establishing a territory，establishing a niche，occupying the niche and five steps—background，aim/ objectives/purpose，method/materials/patients，results/findings and conclusions/ recommendation（Swales，1990；Kanoksilapatham，2005；Hartley，2008；Wallwork，2012），see Table 1.3.

Table 1.3　Move structures of a medical working abstract

Moves	Steps		Structures
Move 1 Establishing a territory	Step 1	Claiming centrality	Give a basic introduction to your research area, which can be understood by researchers in medical discipline (1—2 sentences). Provide more detailed background for researchers in your field (1—2 sentences).
	Step 2	Making topic generalizations	
	Step 3	Reviewing items of previous research	
Move 2 Establishing a niche	Step 1A	Counter-claiming or	State the problem
	Step 1B	Indicating a gap or	
	Step 1C	Question-raising or	
	Step 1D	Continuing a tradition	
Move 3 Occupying the niche	Step 1A	Outlining purposes or	Aims/objectives/purposes
	Step 1B	Announcing present research	
	Step 2	Outlining your methodology	Patients/materials where appropriate
	Step 3	Announcing principal findings	Provide some more information regarding your results (1—2 sentences).
	Step 4	Explaining the implications	Tell the reader the implications of your results (1—2 sentences).

2. Vocabulary for abstracts

（1）Background

a number of studies	It is known that
has reduced	Recent work found large effects of
has been foundational to distinguish	It is widely accepted that
exist(s)	occur(s)
It is important to understand the scope of	have been identified
have developed	often
frequently	have demonstrated...
Few studies in AD have tested	popular
generally	produce(s)
There is a need to identify	recent research
have evolved from...	recent studies
is a common technique	recently
is/are assumed to	recently-developed
is/are based on	A recent randomised trial showed
is/are determined by	...
have transformed treatment approaches...	
is/are influenced by	
is/are related to	
It has recently been shown that	

（2）Aim，purpose and objective

in order to integrate	to examine
was supported	We hypothesized that
to determine whether	to investigate
our approach	our study aims to carry out
to characterize features of	to study
the aim of	have revolutionized the approach to
offers the potential of unveiling novel	with the aim of
to evaluate the utility of	here we test whether
this study to compare	is unknown
the field of precision medicine aims to	was designed to screen for potential
（an）alternative approach	This study examines the association
Thus，it is important to understand the scope of	impractical
a need for	the current study translates methods used in
This is the first（RCT）designed to identify	inaccurate
We aimed to explore	We investigate the interaction
complicated	to characterize
Therefore，we aim to determine	To determine the stability of
desirable	inconvenient
Here，we analyzed the feasibility	We report the feasibility of
disadvantage	This study investigated the feasibility of
Our aim is to advance	It should be possible to
essential	no studies explored
the current study applies expensive	however
This study investigated body mass index	…

（3）Methodology，patients and materials

was/were assembled	was/were modeled
The parent study randomized	was measured and atypical balance was derived
was/were designed to evaluate	using
was defined using	was/were performed
was/were calculated	was/were used to evaluate
was/were randomly assigned to	was constructed by
was/were constructed	Participants completed
are randomized to	was/were recorded
are allocated into	we reanalyzed
was/were applied to	is collected with
was/were set based on	was/were studied
was/were included	The main outcome of this study was to evaluate
The primary outcome measure is	was/were treated
was/were evaluated	had better outcomes with
was/were screened	was/were used
was conducted	Unsupervised analyses identified
We tested this hypothesis in	was used to obtain predicted outcomes
was designed based on	were obtained for likely
Primary outcome was organ support	The assessment is performed
was/were formulated	The predefined primary outcome measure was
were formulated and preregistered	were up-titrated to
was/were measured	has included patients

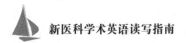
（4） Results，achievement and contribution

caused	was/were achieved
The findings may serve as a novel model for	This predictive relationship survived
decreased	was/were found
interactions significantly predicted	Patients were randomly assigned to training
had no effect	was/were identical
patients were collected and screened from	was/were determined by
increased	was/were observed
It was noted/observed that...	These factors were included in
occurred	was/were obtained
The improvements scaled with	Patients in training set showed
produced	was/were present
were enrolled	was/were unaffected（by）
resulted	revealed
were quantified	provided support for
in was identified	achieve
accurate	indicated strong evidence of
significantly differed between	indicated
better	were similar to
have been recruited	were more strongly associated with
We confirmed	allow
Consistent	was associated with
was supported	improved outcomes for
effective	demonstrate
were statistically significantly worse	ensure
enhanced	guarantee
exact	obtain
improved	validate
new	compare well with
novel	for the first time
There was a significantly	in good agreement
significant	are expected
simple	changed significantly in
suitable	involved in
superior	...

（5） Conclusion，discussion and application

The evidence/These results...	It is thought that
We reported	This work informs
prescriptively predicted higher likelihood of	We conclude that
indicate(s) that	has a good predictive ability for
explain inconsistent results with	We suggest that can/may
mean(s) that	make it possible to
In sum，we provide evidence for	This holds promise for progress
suggest(s) that	potential use
This project represents	These results encourage the use
applicability	relevant for/in

Continued

The results are relevant to	There are substantial causal benefits of
can be applied	could inform
This study demonstrates	are largely stable
can be used	could contribute to
The likely responder statistical paradigm is	will improve
offers insight into	is providing evidence
Our data suggests that	Novel biomarker discovery may enhance
will contribute valuable knowledge concerning	

(6) Limitation, future work and recommendation

a preliminary attempt	future directions
does not account for	needs to be clarified in the future
not significant	future work
slightly	The hypothesis is planned to be tested
Future studies will have to validate our findings	future research related to

Task 7B   Build models and move analysis

1. Build models

You are now required to build models for the working abstracts.

Model 1

Advancing Precision Medicine for Alcohol Use Disorder: Replication and Extension of Reward Drinking as a Predictor of Naltrexone Response

Abstract

Background: 1. Precision medicine aims to identify those patients who will benefit the most from specific treatments. 2. Recent work found large effects of naltrexone among "reward drinkers," defined as individuals who drink primarily for the rewarding effects of alcohol. 3. This study sought to replicate and extend these recent findings by examining whether the desire to drink mediated the effect of naltrexone among reward drinkers.

Methods: 4. We conducted a secondary analysis of a 12-week randomized clinical trial of daily or targeted naltrexone among problem drinkers ($n = 163$), with a focus on 86 individuals ($n = 45$ naltrexone and $n = 41$ placebo) who received daily medication. 5. Interactive voice response technology was used to collect daily reports of drinking and desire to drink. 6. Factor mixture models were used to derive reward and relief phenotypes. 7. Moderation analyses were used to evaluate naltrexone effects, with phenotype as a moderator variable. 8. Multilevel mediation tested average desire to drink as a mediator.

Results: 9. Results indicated 4 phenotypes: low reward/low relief; low reward/high relief; high reward/low relief; and high reward/high relief. 10. There was an interaction between the high reward/low relief subgroup ($n = 10$) and daily naltrexone versus placebo on drinks per drinking day (DPDD; $p = 0.03$), percent heavy drinking days ($p = 0.004$), and daily drinking ($p = 0.02$). 11. As compared to placebo, individuals in the high reward/low relief phenotype who received daily naltrexone had significantly fewer DPDD (Cohen's $d = 2.05$) and had a lower proportion of heavy drinking days (Cohen's $d = 1.75$). 12. As hypothesized, reductions in average desire to drink mediated

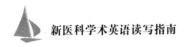

Continued

the effect of naltrexone on average daily drinking among the high reward/low relief drinkers (moderated mediation effect: $p = 0.029$).

Conclusions: **13.** This theory-driven study replicates the empirical finding that naltrexone is particularly efficacious among high reward/low relief drinkers. **14.** Our study brings the field a step closer to the potential of using a precision medicine approach to treating alcohol use disorder.

From Alcohol Clin Exp Res. 2019, 43(11):2395 - 2405, by Katie Witkiewitz et al.

Model 2

Precision Medicine Approach to Alzheimer's Disease: Successful Pilot Project

Abstract

Background: **1.** Effective therapeutics for Alzheimer's disease are needed. **2.** However, previous clinical trials have pre-determined a single treatment modality, such as a drug candidate or therapeutic procedure, which may be unrelated to the primary drivers of the neurodegenerative process. **3.** Therefore, increasing data set size to include the potential contributors to cognitive decline for each patient, and addressing the identified potential contributors, may represent a more effective strategy.

Objective: **4.** To determine whether a precision medicine approach to Alzheimer's disease and mild cognitive impairment is effective enough in a proof-of-concept trial to warrant a larger, randomized, controlled clinical trial.

Methods: **5.** Twenty-five patients with dementia or mild cognitive impairment, with Montreal Cognitive Assessment (MoCA) scores of 19 or higher, were evaluated for markers of inflammation, chronic infection, dysbiosis, insulin resistance, protein glycation, vascular disease, nocturnal hypoxemia, hormone insufficiency or dysregulation, nutrient deficiency, toxin or toxicant exposure, and other biochemical parameters associated with cognitive decline. **6.** Brain magnetic resonance imaging with volumetrics was performed at baseline and study conclusion. **7.** Patients were treated for nine months with a personalized, precision medicine protocol, and cognition was assessed at $t = 0, 3, 6,$ and 9 months.

Results: **8.** All outcome measures revealed improvement: statistically significant improvement in MoCA scores, CNS Vital Signs Neurocognitive Index, and Alzheimer's Questionnaire Change score were documented. **9.** No serious adverse events were recorded. MRI volumetrics also improved.

Conclusion: **11.** Based on the cognitive improvements observed in this study, a larger, randomized, controlled trial of the precision medicine therapeutic approach described herein is warranted.

From Journal of Alzheimer's Disease, 2022, 88(4): 1411 -1421, by Kat Toups et al.

2. Move analysis

Model 1

Move 1 Establish a territory: background

In Sentence 1, the writers provide the aim of the research.

In Sentence 2, the writers provide background factual information.

Move 2 Establish a niche: question raised

In Sentence 3, the writers combine the method, the general aim and the specific aim of the study in one sentence.

Move 3 Occupy the niche: methods, results and conclusions

In Sentences 4—8, the writers summarize the methodology, provide details, and outline materials where appropriate.

In Sentences 9—12, the writers explain what your main result reveals and/or adds when compared to the current literature and indicate the achievement of the study.

In Sentences 13—14, the writers put the results into a more general context and explain the implications.

Model 2

Move 1   Establish a territory: background

In Sentences 1—2, the writers give a basic introduction to your research and review items of previous research.

Move 2   Establish a niche: indicating a gap

In Sentence 3, the writers introduce the background by connecting in some way to what they said in their introductory sentence to indicate the gap.

Move 3   Occupy the niche: purpose, methods, results and conclusions

In Sentence 4, the writers combine the method, the general objective and the specific objective of the study in one sentence.

In Sentences 5—7, the writers provide more detailed methodology and materials.

In Sentences 8—10, the writers explain what the main result reveals and/or adds when compared to the current literature.

In Sentence 11, the writers present the implications of the study.

3. The models rebuilt

The sentence types we have collected can reconstruct basic components of the structure abstract as follows:

Numbers	Components
1	background, objective, aim, purpose, problem, goal
2	methodology, materials, patients, participant
3	results, findings, achievement, contribution
4	implications, applications, discussion, conclusions
5	suggestions, limitations, future work

Task 8   Final assignment: Write a working abstract

Find an example of precision medicine. Search "Precision medicine in oncology" or "Genomics in precision medicine" on the internet, or use a sample provided by your instructor. Write a working abstract about precision medicine, including the basic components.

- Learn as much as you can about the introduction, methodology, findings and conclusions of this sample.
- Write a working abstract for your research.

Further reading

Barlesi, F., Tomasini, P., Karimi, M., et al. (2022). Comprehensive genome profiling in patients with metastatic non-small cell lung cancer: the precision medicine phase II randomized SAFIR02-lung trial. *Clin Cancer Res*. 28(18): 4018-4026.

Cross, C., & Oppenheim, C. (2006). A genre analysis of scientific abstracts. *Journal of documentation*, 62(4), 428-446.

Hartley, J. (2008). *Academic writing and publishing: A practical handbook*. Routledge.

Helland, Å., Russnes, H. G., Fagereng, G. L., et al. (2022). Improving public cancer care by implementing precision medicine in Norway: IMPRESS-Norway. *J Transl Med*. 20(1):225.

Kanoksilapatham, B. (2005). Rhetorical structure of biochemistry research articles. *English for specific purposes*, 24(3), 269-292.

Mattei, Larissa H. Robb, M. D., Lauren, B S, et al. (2022). Enrollment of Individuals from racial and ethnic minority groups in gynecologic cancer precision Oncology trials. *Obstetrics & Gynecology*. 140(4): p654-661.

Neelapu, S. S., Dickinson, M., Munoz, J., et al. (2022). Axicabtagene ciloleucel as first-line therapy in high-risk large B-cell lymphoma: the phase 2 ZUMA-12 trial. *Nat Med*. 28(4):735-742.

Pixberg, C., Zapatka, M., Hlevnjak, M., et al. (2022). COGNITION: a prospective precision oncology trial for patients with early breast cancer at high risk following neoadjuvant chemotherapy. *ESMO Open*. 7(6):100637.

Rodriguez, G. M., Wood, E. H., Xiao, L., et al. Community health workers and precision medicine: a randomized controlled trial. *Contemp Clin Trials*. 2022, 121:106906.

Salager-Meyer, F. (1990). Discoursal flaws in medical English abstracts: A genre analysis per research and text-type. *Text-interdisciplinary journal for the study of discourse*, 10(4), 365-384.

Salager-Meyer, F. (1992). A text-type and move analysis study of verb tense and modality 10distribution in medical English abstracts. *English for specific purposes*, 11(2), 93-113.

Swales, J. M., & Swales, J. (1990). *Genre analysis: English in academic and research*

settings. Cambridge University Press.

Toups，K.，Hathaway，A.，Gordon，D.，et al. (2022). Precision medicine approach to alzheimer's disease：successful pilot project. *J Alzheimers Dis*. 88(4)：1411 – 1421.

Wallwork，A. (2012). *English for academic research: Writing exercises*. Springer Science & Business Media.

Witkiewitz K.，Roos C. R.，Mann K.，et al. (2019). Advancing precision medicine for alcohol use disorder：replication and extension of reward drinking as a predictor of naltrexone response. *Alcohol Clin Exp Res*. 43(11)：2395 – 2405.

Yin，J.，Shen，S.，Shi，Q. (2022). Challenges，opportunities，and innovative statistical designs for precision oncology trials. *Ann Transl Med*. 10(18)：1038.

Unit 2
Reading and Writing an Introduction

In the following units we will discuss how to read and write each part of the move structure of a medical research paper (the introduction, method, results, discussion and conclusion). A well-written introduction section of an original research paper is generally located at the beginning the problem, novelty, and gaps of the current research. A poorly constructed introduction not only discourages the readers from understanding the contents of the paper, but also is likely to be rejected by peer-reviewers. A good introduction is required to be brief, well-referenced, well-organized and introduce the subject, perhaps with a definition or some historical background.

Highlight

In this unit, you will

- Learn vocabulary related to translational medicine and accurate immunology
- Organize move-steps that reflect your introduction writing
- Use suitable expressions and types of sentences to organize a cause-effect essay
- Learn about building an academic vocabulary bank to help you write an introduction
- Write a short cause-effect essay with the move-steps
- Build a model for an introduction
- Write an introduction that includes your move-steps and model

Gearing up

The following passage summarizes the logic patterns of an effective introduction.

It is worth emphasizing the need for a logical path through the literature. All too often an Introduction provides a variety of interesting background facts, but little (or no) logical linking of these. Even experienced researchers sometimes fall into the trap of treating the Introduction as some form of task list: 'I need to have a section that talks about this, and a section about this other thing, and I also need to mention the work of authors X and Y'. What starts life as a list often continues as one. What is missing is a narrative structure that clearly outlines a logical argument. I would therefore discourage authors from initially thinking 'What needs to be in my Introduction', and rather think 'What is the logical argument that the Introduction is trying to make?'

One indicator that an Introduction has become a list of background facts, rather than a logical argument, is the absence of linking conjunctions. For example, conjunctions such as 'However,...' or 'In contrast,...' often highlight where conflicts exist between studies that the current study might redress. Conjunctions such as 'Therefore,...', 'Because of this,...' or 'As such,...' often highlight where a logical extension of an argument-or a hypothesis-is being made, which the study might test. A further indicator that you are failing to outline a logical argument is if your Introduction is still readable when the sentences describing previous studies are omitted. This suggests your discussion of the literature is not being used to shape an argument, but is largely descriptive.

This is not to say that facts cannot appear in the Introduction. Often, concepts need to be defined, a particularly unfamiliar technique briefly outlined or the general importance of a field of study established. However, such statements should be added to a well-thought out shortest logical path (see above) and be kept as brief as possible so that the logical flow of this path is not interrupted.

From Ophthalmic Physiol Opt. 2022, 43(1): 1-3, written by A. J. Anderson

Work in small groups, and discuss the following questions.
1. What are common problems in an introduction?
2. Which logic patterns are mentioned in the passage? How do you identify them?
3. What regular markers for cause and effect relations are mentioned in the passage?
4. How many logic patterns do you know? What are they?

Section 1　Reading

Task 1　Activating background knowledge

Task 1A　Talk about English for medical purpose with your classmates.
1. What is medical English?
2. For what purpose do we learn medical English?
3. What difficulties do you have when reading medical texts?

Look at Table 2.1 and tick your items, then share your answers with your classmates.

Table 2.1 Questionnaire for difficulties in medical text reading

Difficulties in medical text reading	Very easy	Easy	General	Difficult	Very difficult
The goals of medical language and terminology					
The use of metaphor in science					
What makes medical writing sound so medical					
Patterns in medical discourse that signal speculation as well as certainty					
How scientists persuade each other, how they employ scientific rhetoric to argue and support their claims					
How the language and discourse of medicine interact with and influence communities outside medicine and how the culture of those outside communities influences medicine					

Task 1B To help you to read academic medical genre effectively, here are some descriptions in Table 2.2 that you are required to tick.

Table 2.2 Questionnaire for the stages of comprehension in reading medical language（Douglas, 2018）

Stages	YES	NO
Lexical processing enables us to make sense of words		
Syntactic processing interacts with our assigning meaning to words, leading us to comprehend their roles in a sentence		
Journals in the medical sciences have encouraged writers to avoid passive construction for good reason recently		
Prefer actors or concrete objects as grammatical subjects		
Avoid using isolated pronouns as grammatical subjects		
Prefer action verbs		
Avoid using expletives		
Understand how sentences relate to each other: inferential processing		
Put important information in the sentence emphasis position		
Use sequencing for a string of complex or contentious ideas		
Use transitions to tie sentences together		
Grasp how sentences work together to build a coherent statement or argument		

Task 2 Understanding the facts and details

Reading 1 Text theme: Science translational medicine

Task 2A Read the text, and fill in the blank with the proper form of the word in each bracket.

Novel Fhr2 Variants in Atypical Hemolytic Uremic Syndrome: A Case Study of a Translational Medicine Approach in Renal Transplantation
Emma Diletta Stea et al

1. Atypical hemolytic-uremic syndrome (aHUS) is a systemic endotheliosis that is characterized by severe microangiopathy and renal failure, leading to uncontrolled activation of the alternative complement pathway. The causes of this severe kidney disease are genetic abnormalities, mostly of complement genes, and acquired factors abnormalities, most of which affect the binding affinity of the central regulator, factor H, to the cellular surface. The imbalance between complement activators and regulators leads to enhanced lytic complement complex (C5b-9) deposition in the vasculature, _____ (primary) in glomerular blood vessels. Vascular damage drives kidney dysfunction and, therefore, blockade of distal complements and of lytic C5b-9 is the major goal of current therapeutic approaches, for example with eculizumab or ravulizumab.

2. The specific or individual genetic background of patients with aHUS influences the subtle effects of complement action, thus affecting therapeutic responses, recurrence rates, and prognosis throughout the entire process of renal transplantation. In transplant settings, some environmental triggers, such as ischemia-reperfusion injury, acute rejection, and immunosuppressive drugs, _____ induce activation of the complement system and _____ (contributed) to disease recurrence and graft loss.

3. The risk of aHUS recurrence on the allograft _____ (ranging) from less than 20% to more than 90% depending on the patient's genetic background and the therapeutic strategy. Recipients with mutations in the genes encoding circulating complement factors [i.e., C3(C3), factor H, factor I, factor B] have a higher risk of recurrence than patients with genetic variants encoding membrane and local modulators of the complement system, such as cluster of _____ (differentiate) 46 (CD46).

4. Zuber et al. suggested that patients with aHUS can be divided into three different categories according to the risk of post-transplant disease recurrence. Mutations in factor H, rearrangement in factor H/factor H-related (FHR) genes, gain of function mutations in C3 and complement factor B, and a previous history of aHUS recurrence were found to be associated with a high recurrence risk, and this was confirmed Kidney Disease Improving Global Outcomes (KDIGO) working group, which recommends the prophylactic use of eculizumab on the day of transplantation to

prevent overactivation of the complement system. In these puzzle-like scenarios, the discovery of novel genes and of novel risk variants associated to aHUS is of high interest and significance. To determine the most appropriate therapeutic _____ (intervene) in an individual patient, especially in a transplant setting, investigation of the exact genetic background, gene risk haplotypes, and autoimmune factor is extremely helpful, as the prophylactic use of eculizumab, ravulizumab, or plasma therapy remains at clinicians' discretion.

5. Here, we present the first case of a patient with aHUS carrying two novel FHR2 gene variants and with severely reduced plasma levels of FHR2. Eberhardt et al. have shown that FHR2, a novel complements modulator and inhibitor, inhibits C3 convertase and blocks C5b-9 assembly. However, the exact role of FHR2 in complement modulation, in particular how it interact with other FHRs (i.e., multimer formation with FHR1 and FHR5) and with complement components, such as C3, the cleavage products C3b and C3d, and its _____ (involve) in aHUS pathogenesis are still unclear.

6. Faced with a patient who was a candidate for a kidney transplant, we performed a set of functional assays in vitro to determine if extremely low FHR2 plasma levels can influence complement activation and C5b-9 deposition on endothelial cellular surfaces, and, if so, whether or not these effects could be reversed by restoring FHR2 levels or by eculizumab. We then used the results of the in vitro assays to inform and formulate the best therapeutic approach for this specific patient. The in vitro tests showed that extremely low plasma FHR2 levels can induce complement activation and enhance C5b-9 deposition endothelial cells, suggesting that low FHR2 levels can form the basis for aHUS onset. Moreover, both recombinant FHR2 and eculizumab were able to control complement action in the patient's plasma, and to reduce endothelial C5b-9 deposition to a similar degree. Collectively, these findings allowed us to tailor _____ (induce) therapy and maintenance therapy following kidney transplant. This translational approach, based on genetic testing, circulating complement profiling, and functional in vitro experiments, provides a novel framework that is useful to optimize the targeted treatment of complement dysfunction in the clinical setting.

From the Journal Frontiers in Immunology, 2022, 13:1008294

Task 2B Read the text more closely. Decide whether these statements are TRUE (T) or FALSE (F).

1. Atypical hemolytic-uremic syndrome can be relieved by recombinant FHR2 and eculizumab (aHUS).   (   )

2. The causes of this severe kidney disease are vascular damage drives kidney dysfunction.   (   )

3. The prophylactic use of eculizumab on the next day of transplantation is to

prevent overactivation of the complement system.　　　　　(　　)

4. Knowing whether extremely low FHR2 plasma levels can influence complement activation and C5b − 9 deposition on endothelial cellular surfaces is basis of therapeutic approach for this specific patient.　　　　　(　　)

5. Recombinant FHR2 and eculizumab increase endothelial C5b − 9 deposition to a similar degree.　　　　　(　　)

6. Optimizing the targeted treatment of complement dysfunction in the clinical setting needs the results of the in vitro assays of the specific patient.　(　　)

Task 3　Academic literacy skills

Task 3A　Organize the information

Often you will have to record the information when reading texts in order to use it in your writing. Practice in your group, and check your skills of identifying scientific information.

Activity 1　Identify key information

Read the following extracts and identify the main idea of each extract.

Extract 1　Biobanks are biorepositories aimed at the collection, storage, processing, and sharing of human biological samples and associated data for research and diagnosis. Their role is crucial not only for biomarker discovery and validation but pharmaceutical/biotechnology industry. Owing to the unprecedented opportunities provided by big data collection and artificial intelligence, the role of biobanks in cancer research is continuously evolving.

Extract 2　The ERNs, Share4Rare and Rare Barometer are designed to foster people or patient-centric projects. In these programs, citizens/patients play a role beyond that of the traditional research participant. They are treated as equal partners and whose insights, preferences, values, and beliefs are continuously sought and incorporated. Importantly, people-centric projects ensure that the needs and priorities of citizens/patients are addressed

Activity 2　Select and use information

1. Read the following paragraph on Immunology and Congenital Disorders of Glycosylation questionnaire. Identify important information, and check with your partners.

2. Use the information you have selected to write a short comment on this paragraph. You should use your own words as more as possible.

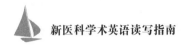
ImmunoCDGQ Attained High Participation, Inclusion Rates and English Version Representativeness

The ImmunoCDGQ (CDG group) and the ImmunoHealthyQ (control group) were initiated by 509 and 954 participants, respectively (Table 1, Fig. 4A, C). Participants had to read and agree to the electronic informed consent to proceed to the questionnaire. In the CDG group, 4 participants did not consent to participate whereas all control participants agreed to take part in the study. The average completion rate, i.e., the percentage of participants who completed the entire questionnaire was below 50% and equivalent between both groups, being of 43.4% (221 out of 509) in the CDG group and of 43.6% (416 out of 954) among controls (Table 1). What differed was the inclusion rate, i.e., the percentage of included participants following the fltering of the inclusion/ exclusion criteria. Questionnaire inclusion rate was much higher in the CDG group (94.6%, 209 out of 221) compared to controls (83.9%, 349 out of 416) (Table 1). Reasons for excluding complete questionnaires among the CDG group included (i) unconfirmed or incomplete CDG diagnosis ($n = 10$) and (ii) strong suspicions of duplicated patient reporting ($n = 2$). In the control group 67 participants were excluded for having a genetic or chronic condition. Regarding the questionnaire language distribution and representativeness, most of the initiated and included ImmunoCDGQ responses were in English, followed by Spanish and then Italian (Fig. 4A, B). Contrastingly, the most represented language in the ImmunoHealthyQ was Portuguese, followed by Italian and English (Fig. 4C, D). Regarding completion and inclusion rates of the different language versions, they varied not only between the control and CDG groups but also amongst themselves (Additional file 1: Tables S5 and S6). The included 209 CDG and 349 control participants were from 31 and 12 countries, respectively. Complete participant demographics are detailed in (Fig. 4E).

From Orphanet J Rare Dis. 2022, 17(1):134, written by R. Francisco et al.

Task 3B Moves in medical English structured introduction

Generally, an introduction contains relevant literature, knowledge background, the gap of current knowledge, the research question or hypothesis, and the methodology used to occupy the gap and respond to the question. Swales and Feak (2004, 2012) describe these characters as "moves" in the various sections of academic articles. Tables 2.3—2.5 show typical "moves" for an introduction.

Table 2.3　Swales' CARS model (Bawarshi & Reiff, 2010)

Move 1		Establishing a territory
	Step 1	Claiming centrality and/or
	Step 2	Makig topic generalization(s) and/or
	Step 3	Reviewing items of previous research
Move 2		Establishing a niche
	Step 1A	Counter-claiming or
	Step 1B	Indicating a gap question-raising or
	Step 1C	Question-raising or
	Step 1D	Continuing a tradition
Move 3		Occupying the niche
	Step 1A	Outlining purposes or
	Step 1B	Announcing present research
	Step 2	Announcing principal findings
	Step 3	Indicating RA structure

Table 2.4　Bunton's modified CARS model for Ph.D. thesis introduction (Bunton, 2001)

Often present	Occasionally present
Move 1: Establishing a territory **STEPS**	
1. Claiming centrality	
2. Making topic generalizations and giving background information	Research parameters
3. Defining terms	
4. Reviewing previous research	
Move 2: Establishing a niche **STEPS**	
1A Indicating a gap in research	
1B Indicating a problem or need	
1C Raising questions	Counter-claiming
1D Continuing a tradition	
Move 3: Announcing the present research(Occupying the niche) **STEPS**	
1. Purposes, aims, or objectives	Chapter structure
2. Work carried out	Research question/hypotheses

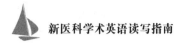

Continued

Often present	Occasionally present
3. Methods	Theorectical positions
4. Materials or subjects	Defining terms
5. Findings or results	Paramaters of research
6. Product of research/model proposed	
7. Significance/justification	Application of product
8. Thesis structure	Evaluation

Table 2.5　Moves in research paper introductions (Swales & Feak, 2012)

Move 1		Establishing a territory
	Step 1	Showing that the general research area is important，central，interesting，problematic，or relevant in some way (optional)
	Step 2	Introducing and reviewing items of previous research in the area (obligatory)
Move 2		Establishing a niche
	Step	Indicating a gap in the previous research or by extending previous knowledge in some way (obligatory)
	In our case，	A niche is a context where a specific piece of research makes particularly good sense.
Move 3		Occupying the niche
	Step 1	Outlining purposes or stating the nature of the present research (obligatory)
	Step 2	Listing research questions or hypotheses (PISF)
	Step 3	Announcing principal findings (PISF)
	Step 4	Stating the value of the present research (PISF)
	Step 5	Indicating the structure of the RP (PISF)

Note：PISF = probable in some fields，but rare in others

Task 4　Building your vocabulary：Match each key word and phrase to its definition.

Word/phrase	Definition
1. potential	**a.** a simplified description of a complex entity or process.
2. induction	**b.** designed to help treat an illness.

Continued

Word/phrase	Definition
3. mechanism	**c.** the inherent capacity for coming into being.
4. presume	**d.** a thin layer of skin or tissue that connects or covers parts inside the body.
5. framework	**e.** developed or used to greatest advantage.
6. alternative	**f.** freedom to act or judge on one's own.
7. discretion	**g.** connected with genes (= the units in the cells of a living thing that control its physical characteristics) or genetics.
8. predominant	**h.** a kind of tissue connecting joints in the body.
9. exploited	**i.** the atomic process that occurs during a chemical reaction.
10. therapeutic	**j.** the chemical processes in living things that change food, etc. into energy and materials for growth.
11. prognosis	**k.** a large cell that is able to remove harmful substances from the body, and is found in blood and tissue.
12. genetic	**l.** relating to the examination and treatment of patients and their illnesses.
13. membrane	**m.** take to be the case or to be true; accept without verification or proof.
14. clinical setting	**n.** an opinion, based on medical experience, of the likely development of a disease or an illness.
15. osteoporosis	**o.** having superior power and influence.
16. metabolism	**p.** the organic processes (in a cell or organism) that are necessary for life.
17. dissected	**q.** allowing a choice.
18. macrophages	**r.** to cut up a dead person, animal or plant in order to study it.
19. metabolism	**s.** a condition in which the bones become weak and are easily broken, usually when people get older or because they do not eat enough of certain substances.
20. bone tissue	**t.** a formal entry into an organization or position or office.

Task 5 Understanding the text moves

Reading 2 Text theme: Accurate immunology

Task 2A Read the text, and fill in each blank with a proper form of the word in the bracket.

Single-cell RNA Sequencing Analysis Dissected the Osteo-immunology Microenvironment and Revealed Key Regulators in Osteoporosis
Yuxin Wang et al

1. Osteoporosis has been predominant to cause arthralgia, joint instability and

especially osteoporotic fracture, which results from aging, osteoarthritis and estrogen deficiency. In the process of osteoporosis, several different types of cells such as macrophages, T lymphocytes and B lymphocytes were stimulated to secrete a variety of proinflammatory chemokines and cytokines. These molecules in turn recruit osteoclast precursors, and mainly act on osteoblasts and marrow stromal cells at the same time to promote their expression level of receptor activator of nuclear factor-κB ligand (RANKL), a vital promotor of osteoclastogenesis. On the surface of osteoclasts and their precursors, RANKL combines with its receptor RANK, triggering activation of numerous intracellular signaling pathways of osteoclast differentiation. However, current approaches for bone study are based on whole cell population of bone instead of individualised cell for bone tissue. This ignores the heterogeneity between single cells and lack of the accurate and resolve to characterize relationships and cross-talks between bone tissue cells. Therefore, it is highly desirable to disclose the mechanism underlying the bone microenvironment and metabolism, thus determining _____ (validity) and promising molecular targets for accurate therapeutic strategy.

2. The scRNA-seq now provides an evolutionary strategy to explore the heterogeneity of complicated tissues and cell-to-cell communication at high _____ (resolve). Other single-cell approaches like Flow cytometry, magnetic activated cell sorting (MACS), immunohistochemistry (IHC) and in situ hybridization (ISH) have a limitation to probe a few selected RNAs. They can only focus on information of the selected RNAs or proteins, while scRNA-seq can provide a broader characterization of the transcriptome profile at higher resolution and with more accuracy. Previous works have revealed the potential mechanisms that decided the osteoclast differentiation process. In the study of Tsukasaki, M. et al., scRNA-seq was performed on murine cells to unveil the transcriptional profiling, reporting the osteoclast fate decision when the cells undergoing osteoclastogenesis in vitro. Based on the results, they identified that CD11c and Cbp/p300-interacting transactivator with Glu/Asp-rich carboxy-terminal domain played a role in triggering final differentiation of osteoclast precursors to become multinuclear osteoclasts. What's more, Hasegawa, T. et al. also discovered that macrophages, isolated from the inflamed synovium on the bare area of arthritic mice and termed as termed arthritis-associated osteoclastogenic macrophages (AtoMs), had the potential to differentiate into osteoclasts. Through the trajectory _____ (analyse) of scRNA-seq, FoxM1 was found to promote the capacity of both human and murine AtoMs to differentiate into osteoclasts, thus _____ (constitute) another possible target for rheumatoid arthritis therapy.

3. In this work, scRNA-seq was utilised to obtained transcriptomic profiles of 19, 102 cells with human femoral head specimens. We have exploited cellular composition of bone tissue cells and restore the different status of osteoclast formation, and cell-specific regulons' modules were determined for dissecting key underlying driving

factors. The zinc finger protein 36, C3H type-like 1 (ZFP36L1) and defensin alpha 3 (DEFA3) were identified as novel bone metabolism-related genes. Meanwhile, _____ (distinctively) subtypes of monocytes, T and B cells in bone microenvironment were also explored to reveal immune landscape of osteoporosis, OC progenitor cells and osteoblast cells. And we further reconstructed the communication cell networks of human femoral head tissues to presume how different types of human femoral head tissue cells work together, which would promote novel insight into cellular landscape of bone metabolism, providing a more _____ (comprehensively) understanding of molecular mechanism and valuable treatment solution of osteoporosis.

From International Immunopharmacology, 2022, 113: 109302

Task 5B   Read the text carefully and decide what the moves are.
1. What's the centrality of the topic in this study?
2. What's the purpose of the research?
3. How did the authors prepare for the present study?
4. What did the authors do to introduce the present study?
5. How did the authors describe the research procedures?

Section 2   Writing

Task 6   Warm-up writing assignment: Write an effective introduction

Task 6A   Verb tense, aspects, voice, signalling language and phraseology in medical English introduction

To use tenses & aspects correctly in an introduction, you are required to focus on three tenses and two aspects, (1) the tenses: the present, the past and the future, (2) aspects: the progressive and the perfect. The two tense pairs by combining tense and aspects to create, e.g., the present simple tense and the present continuous tense; the past simple tense and the present perfect tense, should be differed in the introduction.

1. The simple present tense and the present continuous tense in medical introductions
(1) The simple present tense is used in science writing to express states and habitual activities or state accepted facts and truths, the following are some examples.

> Holistic assessment <u>is</u> an important aspect of providing...
>
> Large B-cell lymphoma <u>accounts for</u> up to 40% of all new diagnoses among...
>
> Breast cancer (BC) <u>is</u> the most common cancer in women, with 2.3 million newly diagnosed cases worldwide per year.

> This strategy <u>facilitates</u> the identification of high-risk patients at the time point of surgery...
>
> Precision oncology trials <u>offer</u> treatment options by application of drugs targeting...
>
> Here we <u>describe</u> the results of the pilot phase of COGNITION...

(2) The present tense is used in citations and paraphrases of information.

> Precision cancer care, an approach that <u>tests</u> a cancer's genetic makeup to identify molecular markers or mutations that can be targeted with treatments, has transformed cancer care and improved cancer survival [1,2].
>
> Adults from low-income households and racial and ethnic minorities with cancer <u>have</u> lower rates of genomic testing [4-6] than more affluent and White adults with cancer.
>
> In these models, surgery-induced natural killer (NK) cell dysfunction <u>plays</u> a key role in determining the outcomes of surgical stress on lung metastases [4-8].
>
> Therefore, perioperative therapies to reverse or prevent NK cell dysfunction <u>have</u> the potential to attenuate the negative sequelae of surgery-induced immunosuppression[3].
>
> Most international guidelines recommend that body mass index (BMI) <u>should</u> be used as a routine measure for diagnosis [3, 10].

(3) The present continuous tense is used to denote action and events that are in the process during a particular specified period of time or at a period of time including the present. This tense seldom occurs in academic medical writing.

> The lesson does a nice job of explaing to the students that they <u>are conducting</u> demonstrations to learn about what causes a linghting strike.
>
> This could start the student's thinking about their grammar when they <u>are doing</u> informal writing outside of their portfolios
>
> Together these findings suggest that enrichment <u>is having</u> a dynamic influence on striatal PNN formation.

2. The simple past tense and the present perfect tense in medical introductions

(1) Most contextual uses of the simple past tense are to denote a single event or state that happened or existed in the past, indicated by past time adverbs.

For example, the precision oncology trial CATCH for patients with advanced/metastatic BC <u>revealed</u> a clinical benefit for about one-third of treated patients.

In our own preclinical animal studies, perioperative arginine-enriched food <u>increased</u> blood arginine levels, <u>improved</u> NK cell recovery, <u>and reduced</u> metastatic burden after surgery.

Recently, AI-assisted endocytoscopy <u>showed</u> an adequate accuracy for $\leqslant$ 5-mm rectosigmoid polyps, achieving $a \geqslant 90\%$ negative predictive value (NPV) for adenomatous histology in a real-time setting.

(2) The present perfect tense combines perfective aspect with the present tense to create for a new complex verb phrase forms and meanings. The past event is considered more relevant to the situation now.

Chimeric antigen receptor T-cell therapies targeting CD19 <u>have demonstrated</u> manageable safety profiles and high efficacy in the treatment of relapsed/refractory B-cell lymphomas, including LBCL, mantle cell lymphoma and follicular lymphoma.

So far, however, this approach <u>has been mainly confined to</u> the palliative setting.

The emergent field of implementation science <u>has generated</u> many insights into the barriers to and facilitators of the effective uptake and deployment of new health technologies.

3. The use and functions of active/passive voice in medical introductions

(1) The passive voice plays an important role in process descriptions. One of the functions in medical introductions is to project an academic indirectness, detachment, and objective.

Remarkably, combining the escape maps with these functional measurements predicts which mutations are selected when spike-expressing virus <u>is grown</u> in the presence of individual antibodies.

All annotation, taxonomy information, and metadata <u>are combined to</u> generate several outputs.

(2) The natural processes without direct human intervention are commonly used to describe by active voice or a mix between active and passive (Swales & Feak, 2012).

Current sequencing techniques <u>require</u> single-cell suspensions for passage through microfluidic or microwell platforms，and the generation of single-cell suspensions from solid tissues requires the enzymatic and mechanical disruption of extracellular matrix and cell-cell contacts.

Regeneration of central nervous system（CNS）myelin <u>involves</u> differentiation of oligodendrocytes from oligodendrocyte progenitor cells（OPC）.

Hi-C <u>exposes</u> unique microchromosome biology Our analyses of the first chromatin contact data for a nonmammalian vertebrate demonstrate broad similarities in chromatin structure across vertebrate macrochromosomes，yet unique features of snake microchromosomes.

4. Signalling language in medical introductions

（1）Sentence connection

① The easiest way to connect sentences is to repeat key nouns frequently from the previous sentence.

<u>Precision oncology trials</u> offer treatment options by application of drugs targeting molecular alterations detected in tumor cells via genomic and/or transcriptomic profiling approaches. For example，<u>the precision oncology trial CATCH</u>（Comprehensive assessment of clinical features and biomarker to identify patients with advanced or metastatic breast cancer for marker driven trials in humans）for patients with advanced/metastatic BC revealed a clinical benefit for about one-third of treated patients.

② The second way is to replace a key noun with the pronoun "it/they" to make the paragraph flow smoothly.

Although <u>CAR T-cell therapy</u> is established for the treatment of relapsed/refractory B-cell lymphomas，<u>its</u> potential when applied as part of first-line therapy for patients at risk of early chemotherapy failure has not been studied

<u>Two additional patients</u> who relapsed did not have evaluable samples at the time of relapse，although <u>they</u> had detectable CAR gene-marked cells in blood at the final time point assessed before relapse.

Although the existence of these interfaces is reflected indirectly in the quantitative μMRI <u>profiles</u> using UTE，<u>they</u> are not directly distinguishable in μMRI SE or GE sequences due to the strong dipolar interaction.

③ The third way is to use transition signals to indicate the relationship between sentences.

<u>For example</u>, longer culture times or the use of HSC expanding reagents prior to editing may drive cells into cycle and increase the probability of cell division with a broken chromosome. (Telling readers that an example of the preceding achievement is coming)

<u>Moreover</u>, loss-of-function experiments demonstrate impaired baroreflex function, attenuated BP rise and decreased sympathetic outflow during DOCA-salt hypertension. (Indicating an additional idea)

When a paired normal was not available, we chose a normal sample from our DLBCL cohort that showed no evidence of tumor in normal contamination and <u>otherwise</u> acceptable QC metrics to remove common germline and potentially remove artifacts resulting from batch effect. (Introducing a choice or alternative).

(2) Choose signal language

From the choices given in the parentheses, choose proper signal language in each group.

① We found that the total deletion load increases, but that the normalized number of unique deletions did not change from younger to older tissue. ____ ____ we observed little change in the size distribution of deletions as well as the relative pools of high-and low-frequency deletions indicating a fairly static spectrum of diversity. (however, in contrast, furthermore)

② Simultaneous multislice in this situation has been used to make tractography possible in routine clinical practice (due to shorter scan times), _____ for visualization of the corticospinal tract and arcuate fasciculus in patients with intra-axial neoplasms, specifically for neurosurgical planning. (however, for example, therefore)

③ Based on these studies, one can propose that Wnt signaling is increased in old animals and that high levels of Wnt are detrimental to organism function. ____ ____ the role of Wnt in the aging process may be more complex, as down-regulation of this pathway can also be detrimental in terms of tissue maintenance. (however, therefore, for example)

④ Unexpectedly, maximum isometric tension was significantly down in the 24-month-old KO mice even though there was significant sparing of muscle mass. _____ the age-associated decrease in tension output was greater in the KO than the WT mice (Fig. S1). (moreover, therefore, for example)

⑤ Finally, it is our practice to remove as much mesh as possible in patients with a mesh complication; therefore, we cannot guarantee that the mesh that underwent analysis was at the exact site of the complication, regardless of whether it was removed for an exposure or pain. _____ the findings of the present study suggest that the 2 major mesh complications (exposure and pain) are associated with a marked proinflammatory response that persists years after mesh implantation. (in conclusion, therefore, however)

⑥ The ill effects of muscle fatigue on proprioceptive sense and altered biomechanics have been reported; _____ muscle endurance training should also be introduced into the rehabilitation program for overhead athletes. (on the other hand, as a result, for example)

5. Phraseology in medical introductions

(1) Establish the importance of the topic for the discipline

> Prognostication is an important **aspect** of clinical decision-making...
> The **key aspects** of the development are presented and discussed in...
> Physicochemical **properties** are **fundamental** to predict...
> Health is a **concept** that is **central** to...
> **Concepts** have a **central** and important place in...
> Neighborhood environments have **received considerable attention** in recent...
> The **fundamental** basis of pyrosequencing is that...
> Perioperative nurses play a **pivotal role** in the successful management of...
> One drug—gabapentin—is **frequently prescribed** in long-term care facilities for...
> Hybrid breeding is **fast becoming** a **key instrument** in...
> Metabolomics has **emerged** as a **powerful** tool for defining...

(2) Review previous research

> There is a **large** and **growing body** of **literature** focusing on the use of oral magnesium...
>
> **Much of the literature** on gender roles and identity is geared toward and written from...
>
> **Over the past decade**, multiple bioinformatics methods and software tools have been developed to identify candidate fusion transcripts from...
>
> **For many years**, research efforts have been directed towards developing such reliable models for more complex materials and composites...
>
> **In recent years** the evolution of new drug and insecticide resistant strains of *Plasmodium* and *Anopheles*...

Historically, the association of the ascending process of the astralogous （ASC） with the tibia is a theropod character that is not found

Computational sequence database mining for diverse CRISPR-Cas systems **has been carried out** by searching microbial genomic

Many recent studies in animals have shown that a large portion of the transcriptome in animals is sex biased （Ranz et al. 2003; Mank et al. 2008）.

It has been demonstrated that Zika virus was introduced to...

（3）Summarize the studies reviewed

Together, **these studies indicate that** CTCF plays an essential role in early neural development and highlight the importance of...

Although **these studies highlight the importance** of neuronal inflammatory and/or stress signaling...

Collectively, **these studies establish** that 78c is a specific, reversible, and uncompetitive CD38i that...

These studies highlight the **important** biological roles uterine EVs/exosomes have...

Taken together **these studies provide a potential** mechanism for initiation of α-syn pathology in...

All of **these studies suggest substantial** communication between...

Together, **these studies demonstrate** that **surfactant** PL plays a critical role in protecting...

These studies provide insight into the liquid demixing of TDP-43 and suggest that small-molecule inhibitors of Tankyrase could be developed...

These studies attribute force generating deficits to baseline reductions in cortical commands, but they do not consider...

These studies have shed light on tissue heterogeneity and provided previously...

（4）Prepare for the present study: Indicate a gap

Far **less** is **known** about how adults...

...**much less** is **known** about how EU-27 Europeans view...

... is **still uncertainty** over when restricting to the complete records is likely to...

However, neither of these processes is well understood...

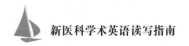

(5) Introduce the present study: State purpose(s)

> The **objective** of this study is to **investigate** the relationship between...
>
> The aim of this **thesis** was to **examine** a population-based cohort of 727 type 1 diabetic patients from...
>
> The present **study aimed** to **investigate** the preparedness of...
>
> The current study **seeks** to **explain** changes in support for violent extremism during the transition to...
>
> The **aim** of the proposed **review** study is mapping **evidence** on the implementation of...
>
> The purpose of this **study** was to **investigate** whether preseason isokinetic strength measures were predictive of future...
>
> The **study** has been **designed** to **investigate** the correlation between clinical and radiological...
>
> This **study** aims to investigate the experiences and insights of nurse educators in order to acquire a **better understanding** of...

Task 6B Literacy skills: Paraphrase and Summary

1. Paraphrase writing

Paraphrasing is to restate the ideas of an original sentence or a text using your own words. Effective paraphrasing is one of the important skills in academic writing to help you to avoid plagiarism, which is intentionally or unintentionally using someone else's words or ideas without acknowledging. Good paraphrasing is rewriting the meaning of the original text and making the paraphrase as long as the original in your own words and sentence structure.

(1) Paraphrase by changing (verbs or nouns)

For example:

> This study **examined** the **stability** of reading **difficulties** from **grades** 2 to 6.
> The study **investigated** the **continuity** of reading **problems** from **batches** 2 to 6.

① Traditional medicine remedies are commonly used for treatment of diverse ailments including bacterial infections.

_____

_____

② Research has found that hypoxia, cold, and drought responses seem to be involved in a plant experiencing hypobaria.

③ Previous studies using murine genetics to study SMAD signaling in the mouse trachea and airway and studies using human tissue have shown that nuclear phosphorylated SMADs are absent from mature tracheal basal cells.

④ Acute neurology is the neurological care that a patient receives in an emergency or urgent care situation.

(2) Paraphrase by changing the verb form
For example:

We further **analysed** the Gene Ontology enrichment of differentially expressed genes and visualized the result in a network map by Cytoscape
The Gene Ontology enrichment of differentially expressed genes and visualized the result in a network map by Cytoscape has been analysed.

① We **observed** a pronounced increase in SPO11-1-oligo density within the CEN180 repeats at the fine-scale in kyp suvh5 suvh6.

② We **examined** regions of chromosomes to get an idea of the local transcriptional landscape structures.

③ We **verified** ddPCR results for the HBD-09 target using endpoint PCR employing forward and reverse primers and gel visualization.

④ We **determined** sufficient sampling by verifying that the effective sample size of key parameters was at least 200 using Tracer v1.7.

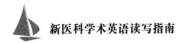

（3）Paraphrase by changing the word class

For example

> Initiating and asking questions allows learners to obtain a better **comprehension** of the content.
>
> <u>Initiating and asking questions allows learners to obtain a better **understanding** the content.</u>

① The repair template included a 3 bp synonymous change to act as a Cas9-blocking mutation and to facilitate the **identification of** gene-corrected iPSC clones by allele-specific PCR.

_____

_____

_____

② Our data indicate an overall **enhancement** of innate immune responses during pregnancy.

_____

_____

③ It is very important to **notice the high variability present** in the dataset，but in these low populated districts，cholera can be seen as a disease with irregular outbreaks，whereas in the former districts cholera exhibits an endemic behavior.

_____

_____

_____

④ Nuclear Magnetic Resonance **is the observation of** the frequency at which magnetic nuclei in molecules come into resonance with an externally applied electromagnetic field.

_____

_____

_____

（4）Paraphrase by changing word order

For example

> This **is quite different from** many other bioinvasions that happen in peoples' backyards.
>
> <u>**There are a number of important differences between** many other bioinvasions that happen in peoples' backyards.</u>

① Injections were **targeted at** the major nuclei of the BF.

_____

_____

② **It is calculated** as the difference of the total number of predicted SCGs and the number of unique SCGs per bin divided by the number of reference SCGs.

_____

_____

③ This finding implies that management policies **aimed at** reducing the future risk of coral bleaching need to consider both "local" nutrient pollution and "global" climate change minimization strategies.

_____

_____

_____

④ It is therefore important now to **confirm** if IL-10 expression is reduced in skeletal muscle from sarcopenic older adults to provide support for its role in muscle loss and frailty in humans.

_____

_____

_____

⑤ There are several pattern recognition receptors (PRRs) function to recognize viruses and foreign nucleic acids (Medzhitov and Janeway, 2000). **These include** the RIG-I like receptors, Rig-I, MDA5, and LGP2, that act as sensors of viral replication within cells, TLR3.

_____

_____

_____

_____

(5) Paraphrase by using synonyms
For example

The other three pre-flight sessions were **considered to be** independent estimates of a putatively stable individual.
considered to be = viewed as/seen as

① Their analysis **only focused on** the bacterial microbiome by mapping reads to reference bacterial genomes. _____

② This amino acid replacement has **arisen** independently multiple times, and in two cases formed lineages of more than 500 sequences. _____

③ The example below **outlines** the general procedure using digital slide images for cell counting. _____

④ We have **provided** novel insights into NIRVS in the genomes of important arbovirus vectors. _____

⑤ Few studies have **examined** sources of individual resilience. _____

⑥ This analysis was **conducted** for each joint and visit separately.

_____

⑦ The first statement **claims** that the values have a frequentist sampling theory interpretation. _____

⑧ They **contend** that hypertension could increase blood-brain-barrier permeability, resulting in an increase in extracellular water.

_____

⑨ The objective of this study is to **assess** the effects of antidepressants on the natural fertility in women. _____

⑩ The same line of results **can be found** in playing positions associated with laterality in handball. _____

（6）Paraphrase by using all these skills

Two direct quotations related to the similar topic are provided as follows:

> The network will facilitate trial readiness through the establishment of an ERN-RND registry with..., thus providing a unique overview of existing genotype-based cohorts. The overall aim of the ERNs is to improve access for patients with RDs to quality diagnosis, care, and treatment....to provide transparency and reassurance to the RD community and the general public. *From Orphanet J Rare Dis Orphanet. 2021, 11: 616569, written by C. Reinhard, et al.*

> Importantly, unresolved challenges may have a strong impact on the further sustainability of ERNs and their ability to realize full potential in addressing huge unmet needs of RD patients and their families.
>
> *From J. Community Genet. 2021, 12(2): 217 –229, written by B. Tumiene, et al.*

Paraphrase:

Several international initiatives have been exploring these e-health and e-research pathways. Among which stand the European Reference Networks（ERNs）, whose primary aim is to serve as virtual care networks connecting medical experts and RD patients across Europe. Also, the ERNs hold great e-research potential（Reinhard, et al., 2021; Tumiene, et al., 2021）.

① The authors propose the use of a structured Practice-Based Clinical Research Network to perform patient-centered outcomes research consistent with the requirements of the pharmaceutical sector in a safe, ethical, and effective manner and congruent with the principles of Good Clinical Practice.（From *Ther Innov Regul Sci*. 2013, 47（3）: 349－55, written by D. A. Robbins, et al.）.

Implementing the innovations proposed by the CDG community is likely to have ethical, legal and social implications associated with the potential donation of patients' clinical and biological material that need to be assessed and regulated...To promote people-centred care for the CDG community, and increase its participation..., it is necessary to create participatory spaces...（*From BMC Health Serv Res*. 2017, *17:682*, *written by C. De Freitas, et al.*）

Your paraphrase:

_____

_____

_____

_____

② The median time to death was 9.6 months. Chemoradiotherapy with TMZ followed by adjuvant TMZ is not more effective than previously reported regimens for the treatment of children with DIPG.（*From Neuro Oncol, 2011, 13:410－6, written by K. J. Cohen*）.

Translation of this knowledge into clinical trials in combination with improved drug distribution methods may eventually lead to more effective treatment of this devastating disease.（*From Cancer Treat Rev, 2012, 38:27－35, written by M. H. Jansen*）.

Your paraphrase:

_____

_____

_____

_____

_____

③ The most prevalent HPV genotypes were HPV 16（35%）, HPV 31（16%）HPV 6（9%）, HPV 58 and 66（7%）, followed by HPV 33（6%）, HPV 18 and 56（4%）, HPV 70 and 45（3%）, HPV 53 and 11（2%）. Currently 1.5% of tested specimens

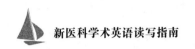

remained unclassified. Multiple infections with at last two different high-risk HPV genotypes were observed in 10% of specimens.(From *Ann Ist Super Sanita*. 2015, 51(3):248 - 51, written by M. F. Coscia, et al.).

This study confirms the effectiveness of antioxidant treatments in the patients affected by BMS, in order to prevent or decrease the onset of oxidative stress and the consequent increased risk of oxidative-related systemic diseases. (*Eur Rev Med Pharmacol Sci* 2012; 16:1218 - 1221, written by M. Tatullo, et al.).

Your paraphrase:

_____

_____

_____

_____

_____

2. Summary writing

Summary writing is a crucial technique both in academic work and in daily life. The students are often required to write a summary after reading a book or paper. Discuss the following tips in Table 2.6 with your partner, and share your views in class.

Table 2.6　Tips for writing a successful summary (Swales & Peak, 2012)

Tips	YES	NO
Scan the text, focus on the subheading or topic sentence of sub-section		
Identify key information, notice your reading techniques		
Read the text, color crucial information or take note		
Write your reflection or ideas concerning about original key information		
Chain the key support points for the key topic consisting of minor details		
Utilize your own lexical and sentence structure		
Include the topic and main supporting points		
Read through your summary again, make your changes royal, appropriate and accurate		

Sumarize each of the following passages

　　Original passage

　　　　It can be difficult to assess the true efficacy of interventions in clinical trials. In phase Ⅲ trials in MS, the traditionally used primary clinical outcome measures are the Expanded Disability Status Scale and the relapse rate.... These secondary outcome measures are often primary outcome measures in phase Ⅱ trials in MS. Despite several limitations, the traditional clinical measures are still the mainstay for assessing treatment efficacy. Newer and potentially valuable outcome measures increasingly used or explored in MS trials are, clinically, the MS Functional Composite and patient-reported outcome measures, and on MRI, brain atrophy and the formation of persisting black holes. Several limitations of these measures have been addressed and further improvements will probably be proposed. Major improvements are the coverage of additional functional domains such as cognitive functioning and assessment of the ability to carry out activities of daily living. The development of multidimensional measures is promising because these measures have the potential to cover the full extent of MS activity and progression...(Source: *CNS Drugs*. 2017, 31:217 - 236, written by van Munster & Uitdehaag).

Summary

Clinical tests require the designation of a basic finding measure on which treatment efficacy can be identified. The findings of the most popular clinical rest consist of the frequency of clinical relapses and deterioration on the Kurtzke Expanded Disability Status Scale (van Munster & Uitdehaag, 2017)

Passage One

Combination of particular clinical [relapses and Expanded Disability Status Scale (EDSS) change] and MRI (lesions and corpus callosum volume change) parameters in the first year was able to predict disability progression.

...NFL levels appear to reflect acute and chronic axonal damage, thus showing an association with relapses and EDSS progression.

...The third sub-study assessed the effectiveness of DMTs on relapses and disability measured with EDSS in the Czech Republic, comparing results from 2007 and 2015. The analysis showed that the number of relapses was associated with a higher risk of progression. Treatment with second generation DMTs was associated with a lower risk of both relapses and progression to EDSS 4.

...NFL levels appear to reflect acute and chronic axonal damage, thus showing an association with relapses and EDSS progression.

The analysis includes three sub-studies, the first of which showed a steep decline in utility at higher EDSS levels, which might suggest room for improvement with respect to treatment...

...Cognitive impairment indicates disease activity or progression and should of course be prevented. However, pure cognitive relapses are controversial at this time. Moreover, transient cognitive decline has been observed at times of increased CNS inflammation.

...Annual re-assessments should follow with the same instrument to detect acute disease activity, to assess for treatment effects or relapse recovery, to evaluate progression of cognitive impairment, and/or to screen for new-onset cognitive problems.

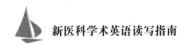
(From Ther Adv Neurol Disord. 2020，13:1756286420975223，written by T. Berger，et al.)

Your summary： _____

_____

_____

_____

_____

Passage Two

Polycystic ovary syndrome (PCOS) is a common heterogeneous endocrine disorder characterized by irregular menses, hyperandrogenism, and polycystic ovaries....Risk factors for PCOS in adults includes type 1 diabetes, type 2 diabetes, and gestational diabetes....Studies show that women with PCOS are more likely to have increased coronary artery calcium scores and increased carotid intima-media thickness. Mental health disorders including depression, anxiety, bipolar disorder and binge eating disorder also occur more frequently in women with PCOS....Recent data suggest that letrozole and metformin may play an important role in ovulation induction. Proper diagnosis and management of PCOS is essential to address patient concerns but also to prevent future metabolic, endocrine, psychiatric, and cardiovascular complications. *(From Clin Epidemiol. 2013,6:1 - 13，written by S. M. Sirmans & K. A. Pate)*

Your summary： _____

_____

_____

_____

_____

_____

Passage Three

Following two decades of more than 400 clinical trials centered on the "one drug, one target, one disease" paradigm, there is still no effective disease-modifying therapy for Alzheimer's disease (AD). The inherent complexity of AD may challenge this reductionist strategy....we consider AD pathobiology, disease comorbidity, pleiotropy, and therapeutic development, and construct relevant endophenotype networks to guide future therapeutic development. Specifically, we discuss six main endophenotype hypotheses in AD: amyloidosis, tauopathy, neuroinflammation, mitochondrial dysfunction, vascular dysfunction, and lysosomal dysfunction. We further consider how this endophenotype network framework can provide advances in computational and experimental strategies for drug-repurposing and identification of new candidate therapeutic strategies for patients suffering from or at risk for AD. We highlight new opportunities for endophenotype-informed, drug discovery in AD, by exploiting multi-omics data. Integration of genomics, transcriptomics, radiomics, pharmacogenomics, and interactomics (protein-protein interactions) are essential for successful drug discovery. We describe experimental technologies for AD drug discovery including human induced pluripotent stem cells, transgenic mouse/rat models, and population-based retrospective case-control studies that may be integrated with multi-omics in a network medicine methodology. (*From Med Res Rev. 2020, 40(6):2386–2426, written by J. Fang et al.*)

Your summary: _____

_____

_____

_____

_____

_____

Task 6C   Cause and effect

1. Cause/effect conjunctive words and phrases

(1) Identify cause/effect conjunctive words and phrases

Discuss with your partner, match the eight parts in Column A to the correct parts in Column B

Column A	Column B
① Our finding of improvement relative to baseline would likely reveal even greater improvement if compared to a control group,	a. **resulted from/was the result of** the injections that included the CeM, supporting the concept of the continuity of these areas found in cytoarchitectural and histochemical work.
② In the case of TRIM28, weak binding to young retrotransposons is known	b. **since/because** decline rather than stability is the observed natural course of MCI and early dementia
③ Our investigation of early events during disease initiation	c. **to result from** them escaping KZNF recognition due to sequence divergence
④ The highest numbers of labeled cells in the SLEAc **resulted from** the injections that included the CeM, supporting the concept of the continuity of these areas found in cytoarchitectural and histochemical work	d. **due to/of because of** dystrophin-deficit has identified poor sarcolemmal repair as an early consequence of dystrophin deficit

Continued

Column A	Column B
⑤ We therefore conclude that the defects in 40S ribosomal subunit production caused by the depletion of human PDCD2 are unlikely to be	e. **as a result of/as consequence of**/the 3$'$ to 5$'$ directionality of mRNA editing.
⑥ We expect a large proportion of intermediates to be amplified by these primer pairs	f. **the consequence of/the effect of** a role of PDCD2 in controlling the expression of ribosome biogenesis genes.
⑦ Two specimens were excluded from subsequent analysis	g. **for** several reasons
⑧ PDPN was chosen as a stromal marker for immunohistochemistry	h. **owing** to low tumor purity as estimated by FACETS analysis.

(2) Recognize cause conjunctive words and phrases

Underline the part of the sentence that states a cause, and bracket the cause conjunctive words and phrases.

E.g. RNA Structure Preferences of RBPs (since) potential RBP binding sites in the transcriptome exist in a variety of structural conformations, and structure is known to impact RBP binding and regulation.

① Due to the considerable admixture in the MW group, we selected a clustering coefficient (Q) cut-off$\geqslant$0.7 for assigning genotypes to a specific cluster.

② We examined whether eNAMPT in the plasma is protected from the protease treatment because of its localization within the EVs.

③ Emerging viral pathogens have caused numerous epidemics and several pandemics over the last century.

④ Currently, there is no clinical indication to separately identify these tumors because BRCA1-and BRCA2-deficient tumors are similarly sensitive to PARP inhibition.

⑤ These distributions show the same results from the regression coefficients.

⑥ These strain turnovers may be the result of spore blooms from a pre-existing cocktail of distantly related strains.

⑦ **As** the study of mitochondrial function in vivo was the purpose of this study, the elasticity coefficient of energy supply was determined under low contraction activity.

⑧ It is commonly believed that hair cell loss that occurs as result of exposure to a pure-tone or narrowband stimulus will result in a discrete band of HC loss.

⑨ These interactions might suggest a reason for the loss of key subunits of the electron transport chain, as the system might preferentially target these subunits, reducing the expression of these proteins, rather than degrading intact, yet dysfunctional mitochondria.

(3) Identify cause/effect conjunctive words and phrases

Discuss with your partner, match the eight parts in Column A to the correct parts in Column B

Column A	Column B
① Prior to MRI examination all participants were fully informed and voluntary jaw movements were calibrated using an instruction video with the same duration as the MRI acquisition	a. **so** they provide a lower level of evidence than experimental studies
② One limitation in the study of gene-diet interactions is that most of the studies are observational	b. **the reason for** migration defect according to the pattern and the region of these two disorder groups of PGCs' movement
③ We should try to find the candidate somatic cells that may be	c. **As a result,** the volunteers were able to move their jaw in a prescribed manner consisting of a homogeneous cycle of maximum opening and closing of the mouth with 10 s duration each
④ Inhibition of HA synthesis	d. **resulted in** loss of CD44 membrane motility
⑤ Moreover, these neuroanatomical changes	e. **the cause of** severe disease and death
⑥ Infections which were once treatable are becoming more and more	f. **had an effect** on overall functional connectivity and network efficiency
⑦ Furthermore, our RNA population model predicts that long non-coding RNAs containing repetitive sequences form networks in local regions	g. **thus** allowing the preferential PCR amplification of molecules bearing an appropriate deletion
⑧ This step consists of targeted endonucleolytic digestion of templates to selectively digest wild-type molecules	h. **thereby** restricting their migration to the cytoplasm
⑨ Most studies of compensatory neural mechanisms in aging use region-specific analyses which bias toward describing local but not age-related global changes	i. **consequently,** they largely ignore the wider neural changes that take place in aging, except insofar as they are related to frontal function
⑩ In estimating latent constructs of cognitive ability, the use of a greater number of indicators in generally preferred	j. **hence** our decision to use subtests with substantive overlap as indicators in multiple models

(4) Recognize effect conjunctive words and phrases

Underline the part of the sentence that states an effect, and bracket the effect conjunctive words and phrases

For example

CTCF helps maintain and form TAD boundaries; (consequently), altering CTCF binding often leads to functional gene expression changes, e. g., oncogenic gene expression in gliomas.

① The selection we observe by comparing Bronze Age and modern samples, therefore, represents only a portion of the total selection.

② From our initial prioritization screen, we confirmed drug sensitivity for a subset of compounds using a tumoroid-formation assay, thus validating our screening method.

③ The throughput and read lengths for these third-generation sequencing technologies continue to improve; as a result, these technologies are increasingly being used to sequence human genomes.

④ Assembly of the reads derived from all three technologies resulted in complete sequences for all 16 yeast chromosomes, as well as the mitochondrial chromosome, in one step.

⑤ The bin size used for binarizing data affects the prediction results, particularly on the predictive power of histone modifications.

⑥ Our framework was therefore also trained to predict the probability of a patient having one or more of several pathologies.

⑦ NCBI genome files frequently do not indicate the source habitat from which viruses or hosts were isolated, so habitat information curated for microbial genomes at Integrated Microbial Genomes was used to generate a list of genera that were isolated from marine habitats.

⑧ This allowed us to accurately determine the overall mutation burden for each patient and detect distinct mutation signatures in highly mutated tumors, thereby identifying patients who stood to benefit from immunotherapy.

2. Use cause/effect conjunctive words and phrases

(1) Use the cause or effect conjunctive word or phrase to form a new sentence by jointing the sentences together.

For example

They are important in limiting the abundance of their hosts.

They can significantly impact the processes and ecosystem functions that prokaryotes carry out.

(thus) They are important in limiting the abundance of their hosts, **thus** they can significantly impact the processes and ecosystem functions that prokaryotes carry out.

① We used an initial threshold of 0.05 rather than 0.

There are no site preferences of 0 in these data sets, and DMS studies are known to under sample the lethal fraction.

(since) _____

② Viruses and hosts can share genes or short sequence elements
   Horizontal gene transfer, the sharing of short regions used in CRISPR defense
   systems, or integration sites used by proviruses.
   (due to) _____

   _____

③ We evaluated an immune compromised model of breast cancer metastasis to
   bone employing intracardiac delivery of MCF-7, ER + cells that cluster with
   the luminal A breast cancer subtype50.
   _____ We believe this is due to persistent immunogenicity of ffluc and eGFP,
   even in animals engineered to express these xenogens at an embryonic stage.
   (consequently) _____

   _____

④ The historical view of mammalian diversification presented by the short fuse
   model often contains broad confidence intervals.
   The short fuse model, through association, is ultimately tied to this
   shortcoming in the molecular clock.
   (as a result) _____

   _____

⑤ We investigated potential pathways related to the hormone leptin, which
   decreases appetite and is a proinflammatory adipokine.
   Hematopoietic niche profiling indicated that LepR + stromal cells relay
   exercise effects.
   (hence) _____

   _____

⑥ The important role they play in the biological processes of a cell.
   Intracellular electric fields are of great interest.
   (because of) _____

   _____

⑦ Our method weighs each nonsynonymous mutation in the human exome
   differentially.
   Our method compares the nucleotide context around each genomic position in
   the human exome with the observed number of mutations at that position.
   (thereby) _____

   _____

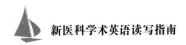

⑧ We can calculate the significance for each observed region r, by comparison with the null area distribution.

We can calculate the significance for each observed region r, by comparison with the null area distribution.

(therefore)_____

_____

_____

⑨ Mild symptoms and many are asymptomatic.

Available data suggest that most Zika virus infections.

(cause-verb)_____

_____

⑩ The additionally found injuries varied from nothing (patient discharged home) to additional observation in the hospital.

The actions undertaken by the trauma team.

(as a result of)_____

_____

(2) Write a cause and effect paragraph

Choose one of the topics related to new medical study and write a paragraph that discusses it in terms of cause and effect.

Precision medicine

Precision medicine and targeted therapies

Precision medicine and obesity

Precision medicine and triple-negative

Precision medicine and radiogenomics

Precision medicine and public health

Precision medicine in oncology

Precision oncology is rapidly reshaping cancer care

The advent of precision medicine in oncology

Functional precision medicine approach to guide treatments

Science translational medicine

Accurate immunology

The accurate measurement of variations in the human immune system

Accurately selecting and evaluating immunotherapies

Cancer systems immunology

Immunology and individuality

Task 7   Writing task: Build a model

Task 7A   Common models and vocabulary in medical introductions

1. Common models of introductions

An outline of scientific writing in Task 2 shows that several models have been presented on how to organize an introduction to a research paper. The problem-solution model of introductions was developed in 1979. Zappen (2019) analyzed the series of sub-contexts including goal, current capacity, problem, solution, and criteria for evaluation. Another common model proposed is Swales's CARS model, which mainly focuses on three moves, that is, establishing a territory (the situation), establishing a niche (the problem), and occupying a niche (the solution). This model can be expanded to Move 4 to explain the arrangement of the paper (Swales & Najjar, 1987; Swales & Feak, 2012). Kanoksilapatham (2005) modified Swale's model of instructions as follows.

Move 1: Announcing the importance of the field	Step 1: Claiming the centrality of the topic
	Step 2: Making topic generalizations
	Step 3: Reviewing previous research
Move 2: Preparing for the present study	Step 1: Indicating a gap
	Step 2: Raising a question
Move 3: Introducing the present study	Step 1: Stating purpose(s)
	Step 2: Describing procedures
	Step 3: Presenting findings

Move 1   Announcing the importance of the field

   Step 1: Claiming the centrality of the topic

> Inflammation likely **plays an important role in** anesthetic hypersensitivity.
>
> Therefore it is plausible that neutrophils **play a key role in** the inflammatory mechanisms seen in sarcopenia and frailty.

   Step 2: Making topic generalizations

> Vascular aging is central to cardiovascular disease, and growing evidence suggests the process **is characterized** not only by changes in extracellular matrix proteins but also by aging of the cells resident in the artery wall.

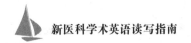

NSIP **is characterized** histologically by varying degrees of interstitial inflammation and fibrosis that are temporally and morphologically homogeneous.

Step 3：Reviewing previous research

The different outcomes of these two tests were unexpected, as we have previously observed that chronic rapamycin treatment **induces** both glucose and pyruvate intolerance due to increased...

We previously emphasized that when dealing with energy balance the accurate calculation of mitochondrial affinity for ADP **requires** the determination of the phosphorylation rate dependenc...

Move 2 Preparing for the present study

Step 1：Indicating a gap

The diagnostic performance of the scale **has not been** reported.

This suggests that neutral amino acids may be particularly important in lysosomal control of mitochondrial function, but the underlying mechanism of this connection is currently **unclear**.

Step 2：Raising a question

Our aim here was to answer key practical **questions** regarding the application of hippocampal volume as a screening tool in aMCI clinical trials.

Many important **questions** remain unanswered: To what extent are regulatory elements functionally conserved across primates?

Move 3 Introducing the present study

Step 1：Stating purpose(s)

This study **was designed to evaluate** key correlates of ferroptosis in the male germline in response to oxidative stress, **explore** the involvement of ALOX15 in this process and **examine** developmental differences in cell death decisions in the testis.

The purpose of **this study was to investigate** whether age-related differences in cortical brain structure accounted for age-related reductions in SWA in a large sample of adolescents.

Step 2: Describing procedures

In this study, we **investigated** how replication is perturbed in BRCA1-deficient cancer cells treated with multiple doses of cisplatin, a crosslinking agent frequently used to treat ovarian cancers.

We therefore **investigated** the ability of MCL-1 deletion to suppress MMTV-PyMT tumour growth when the downstream apoptotic effectors BAX/BAK were reduced.

Step 3: Presenting findings

Our results show that the comparison of matched phylogenetic sets of genomes will be an increasingly powerful strategy for understanding mammalian biology.

In the present study, **we show** that global ischemia induces a transient increase in mTOR phosphorylation at S2448, but suppresses mTOR abundance and functional activity in selectively vulnerable CA1 neurons.

2. Vocabulary for medical introductions

（1）Establishing significance

This article considers the role of the **key** informant **technique** as a qualitative research method and examines the potential contribution of the approach to health care research.

Acute stroke is a **leading cause** of morbidity and mortality in the...

Major issue is optimal anticoagulation in patients with atrial fibrillation and renal disease warranting balance between risks of...

Meta-analyses have become an increasingly **popular method** of drawing conclusions when there are multiple publications addressing a particular topic.

One such technique, deep learning (DL), has become a remarkably **powerful tool** for image processing in recent years.

Our patient had an unusual **rapid rise** in parasite but susceptible to intravenous artesunate.

Organometallic chemists have synthesized a **remarkable variety** of new structural types.

Environmental pollution of heavy metals is increasingly becoming a problem and has become of **great concern** due to the adverse effects it is causing around the world.

There is **growing interest** in the field of psychobiotics，which are probiotics that confer a mental health benefit when ingested.

The review has discussed the **key role** that nurses **play** in the process but warrants more research in the area.

（2）Verbs often used in medical introductions

This was sufficient to **achieve** transduction in the majority of cells with little to no toxicity as assessed by cell division and viability.

Decreased transmission fitness **was demonstrated** for twenty-three mutations，including...

While our profiling analysis described above **focused on identifying** tripeptide stalling motif, we were also able to identify pausing motifs at...

Interestingly，serine restriction **has been shown to** slow cancer progression in tumor-bearing mice.

This measure **was interpreted** as the variety of timing patterns in which the data series pair was coupled.

Correspondence in transposcriptome **has been proposed** as a metric for comparison of cultured human PSC lines to in vivo counterparts.

Changes in medical care for each patient **were reported in** structured self-administered questionnaires completed by the physician who ordered rWGS.

The Thiel embalming technique **was developed** as an alternative preservation technique that maintains tissue pliability, flexibility, and color.

Melting points of the identified compounds were **determined** in open capillary tubes on a Electrothermal melting point apparatus MEL-TEMP and are uncorrected.

While our profiling analysis **described** above focused on identifying tripeptide stalling motifs, we were also able to identify pausing motifs at the dipeptide level in our profiling data.

Although this topic has been much **debated** in the single-cell research community, to our knowledge it has not been previously carefully addressed.

Moreover, tag density in...experiments has been **correlated** to TF affinity, and are also power-law distributed, at least for...

The combined organic layers were dried over sodium sulfate, filtered and **concentrated** under reduced pressure.

Each species listed in the dataset is **categorised** according to its degree of woodiness and climbing strategies.

Task 7B   Build models and move analysis

1. Building models

(1) A typical model of introduction

The introductory paragraph of the essay is like a funnel or an inverted pyramid, from broadest to specific topic by narrowing down. A typical model of introduction used in biomedical paper is highlighted in Figure 2.1(Bahadoran et al, 2018)

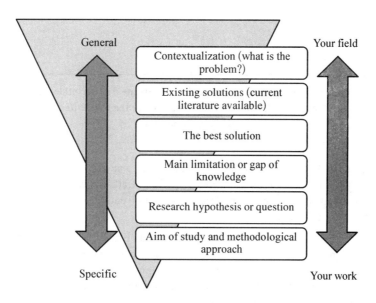

Figure 2.1   **Sequential structure of a typical introduction** (Bahadoran et al, 2018)

(2) Revised Create-A-Research-Space (CARS) Model (Swales, 2004; Sheldon, 2011)

Move 1   Establishing a territory (citations required)

① Reporting conclusion of previous studies

② Narrowing the field

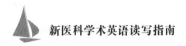

③ Writer's evaluation of existing research

④ Time-frame of relevance

⑤ Research objective/process previous studies

⑥ Terminology/definitions

⑦ Generalising

⑧ Furthering or advancing knowledge

Move 2　Establishing the niche（citations possible）

① Indicating a gap

② Adding to what is known

③（optional）Presenting positive justification

Move 3　Presenting the present work（citations possible）

①（obligatory）Announcing present work descriptively and/or purposively

②（optional）Presenting Research Questions or hypotheses

③（optional）Definitional clarifications

④（optional）Summarising methods

⑤（PISF）Announcing principal outcomes

⑥（PISF）Stating the value of the present research

⑦（PISF）Outlining the structure of the paper

（3）Build models

Model 1

**SARS-CoV-2 mRNA Dual Immunization Induces Innate Transcriptional Signatures,
Establishes T-Cell Memory and Coordinates the Recall Response**
Ι. Papadatou et al

Introduction

1. Since December 2019, severe acute respiratory syndrome coronavirus 2（SARS-CoV-2）has caused a global pandemic, resulting in more than 6 million deaths. 2. Vaccines against SARS-CoV-2 that elicit protective immune responses are crucial to the prevention of the morbidity and mortality caused by SARS-CoV-2 infection.

3. The development of highly effective vaccines is closely tied to the induction of robust and long-live dimmunological memory. 4. Although humoral response to SARS-CoV-2 mRNA vaccines has been extensively reported, studies on other components of the immune response to immunization have been scarce, and the mechanisms that determine the induction, the magnitude and the durability of the mRNA vaccine-induced immunity remain to be elucidated.

5. Moreover, mRNA vaccines against SARS-CoV-2 have demonstrated up to 95% efficacy in preventing severe COVID-19. 6. Despite the proven efficacy, the conferred immunity is short-lived, and the identifications of individuals who respond poorly to vaccination suggests a variability in the vaccine-induced immune response. 7. Therefore, the identification of biomarkers that can detect vaccinated individuals who will mount suboptimal responses is crucial for the optimization of tailored vaccination policies.

Continued

8. In this study, we utilized a systems vaccinology approach in order to comprehensively profile the BNT162b2-induced immune response, investigating both innate and adaptive immunity, and to identify early predictive markers for subsequent recall responses.

From Vaccines 2023, 11(1), 103

Model 2

Development of Gut-Selective Pan-Janus Kinase Inhibitor
TD-1473 for Ulcerative Colitis: A Translational Medicine Programme

William J. Sandborn et al

Introduction

1. Oral Janus kinase [JAK] inhibitors offer a promising treatment option for patients with moderate to severe ulcerative colitis [UC]. **2**. The JAK family comprises four tyrosine kinases, JAK 1-3 and tyro-sine kinase 2 [TYK2], which associate with intracellular domains of the class I and II cytokine receptor superfamily. **3**. Upon binding their cytokine ligands, these receptors activate specific JAK pairings, resulting in phosphorylation-mediated activation of signal transducer and activator of transcription [STAT] proteins, which regulate expression of genes that drive immune cell activation. **4**. The JAK proteins thereby mediate proinflammatory responses to cytokines implicated in UC, including interleukin [IL]-6, IL-23, IL-13, IL-15 and interferon [IFN]γ.2

5. Tofacitinib, a systemically active pan-JAK inhibitor, is approved for induction and maintenance therapy for patients with moderate to severe UC. **6**. However, tofacitinib use is associated with systemic adverse events [AEs]. Reductions in leukocyte subset numbers, serious and/or opportunistic infections, elevations in low-density lipoprotein [LDL] cholesterol, non-melanoma skin cancer and other neoplasms have been observed in patients receiving chronic tofacitinib treatment. **7**. In an ongoing safety trial, pulmonary embolism and death were reported in patients with rheumatoid arthritis taking tofacitinib 10 mg twice daily. **8**. Based on these data, a recent black box warning was issued, and tofacitinib use for UC in the USA is now restricted to patients who have failed tumour necrosis factor [TNF] antagonists. **9**. Despite early results suggesting enhanced efficacy of tofacitinib 15 mg dosed twice daily in Phase 2 and 3 induction clinical trials for UC, tofacitinib 15 mg was not pursued further due to safety signals. **10**. Thus, the currently approved induction [10 mg twice daily] and maintenance [5 or 10 mg twice daily] doses of tofacitinib3 may not achieve maximal efficacy.

11. These data provided proof-of-concept for the potential therapeutic value of a gut-selective JAK inhibitor in patients with UC. **12**. To capture the efficacy of JAK inhibition in UC treatment while minimizing systemic toxicity, we designed TD-1473 as a novel, orally administered, gut-selective pan-JAK inhibitor. **13**. The goal of TD-1473 treatment is to inhibit inflammatory bowel disease [IBD]-related proinflammatory cytokine signalling locally in the gastrointestinal tract with minimal systemic exposure. **14**. Here we report the results of a preclinical and translational medicine programme describing the preclinical pharmacology, pharmacokinetics [PK], efficacy results and safety profile for TD-1473 from preclinical studies, a first-time-in-human [FTIH] Phase 1 study in healthy subjects, and a first-in-patient Phase 1b study in patients with moderately to severely active UC.

From Journal of Crohn's and Colitis, 2020, 1202-1213

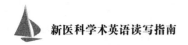

2. Move analysis: Analyze the move structures of the above two models

Model 1

In Sentence 1, the writers establish the importance of this research topic.

In Sentence 2, the writers do the same as in Sentence 1, they provide general background for the reader, suggest why it is important and of interest and/or give some brief historical background.

In Sentence 3, the writers make topic generalizations.

In Sentence 4, the writers describe the general problem area and future research direction, and outline the accepted state and the problem to be resolved.

In Sentence 5, the writers state the achievements of previous research, and announce/preview the main results of the work.

In Sentence 6, the writers indicate the current limitations and state purpose of the research, and state the major objectives, i.e., how to fill the gap.

In Sentence 7, the writers emphasize the purpose of the research again.

In Sentence 8, the writers describe the procedures of the research.

Model 2

In Sentence 1, the writers claim the centrality of this research topic by showing that the general research area is important, central, interesting, problematic or relevant in some way.

In Sentence 2, the writers further provide different classes of materials.

In Sentences 3 – 4, the writers make topic generalizations.

In Sentences 5 – 6, the writers further explain the detailed information of the research and the physical condition of patients in the research using terminology and definitions to underline specific lexis and concepts.

In Sentence 7, the writers review the previous research.

In Sentence 8, the writers indicate limitation of previous research and narrows the focus of the research through increasing specificity.

In Sentence 9, the writers present the general findings of the research.

In Sentences 10, the writers describe the limitations of the method reported in the paper.

In Sentence 11, the writers describe benefits of the research.

In Sentences 12 – 13, the writers state purposes of the research and the benefits of the material.

In Sentence 14, the writers generalize and describe the significance, furthering or advancing knowledge of the research.

3. The models rebuilt

The sentence types we have collected can reconstruct basic components of the structured introduction.

Numbers	Components
1	Establishing a territory (citations required) or the importance of the field (1) Reporting background facts/information or conclusion of previous studies; (2) Narrowing the field; (3) Writers' evaluation of existing research; (4) Time-frame of relevance; (5) Research objective/process previous studies; (6) Defining the terminology/definitions in the title/key words; (7) Generalising the present problem area/current research focus; (8) Furthering or advancing knowledge
2	Previous and/or current research and contributions
3	Establishing the niche (citations possible) (1) Locating a gap in your field; (2) Adding to what is known; (3) (optional) Presenting positive justification
4	Presenting the present work (citations possible) (1) (obligatory) Announcing present work descriptively and/or purposively; (2) (optional) Describing research questions; (3) Presenting the prediction to be tested; (4) (optional) Definitional clarifications; (5) (optional) Summarising methods; (6) Announcing principal outcomes; (7) Stating the thesis statement and the value of the present research; (8) Outlining the structure of the paper

Task 8   Final assignment: Write an effective introduction

Find a paper on translational medicine. Search "Science translational medicine or "Accurate immunology" on the internet, or use the sample provided by your instructor. Write an effective introduction about translational medicine, describing the development in the field.

- Learn as much as you can about the background, previous studies and potentials of translational medicine. Remember to use reliable sources to paraphrase and summarize the information

- Provide the importance, values, gap and definition of the translational medicine

- In the introduction to your essay, apply logic patterns and move structures what you have learned.

Further reading

Anderson, A. J. (2023). Writing an introduction to a scientific paper. *Ophthalmic Physiol Opt*. 43(1):1-3.

Bahadoran, Z., Jeddi, S., Mirmiran, P., et al.(2018). The principles of biomedical scientific writing: Introduction. *Int J Endocrinol Metab*. 16(4):e84795.

Bonizzi, G., Capra, M., Cassi, C., et al. (2022).The road to successful people-centric research in rare diseases: the web-based case study of the Immunology and Congenital Disorders of Glycosylation questionnaire (ImmunoCDGQ). *Orphanet J Rare Dis*. 17(1):134.

Douglas, Y., & Grant, M. B. (2018). *The Biomedical Writer: What You Need to Succeed in Academic Medicine*. Cambridge: Cambridge University Press.

Fried, T., Foltz, C., Lendner, M., et al. (2019). How to write an effective introduction. *Clin Spine Surg*. 32(3):111-112.

Jawaid, S. A., Jawaid, M.(2019). How to write introduction and discussion. *Saudi Journal of Anaesthesia*, 13(Suppl 1):S18-S19.

Papadatou, I., Geropeppa, M., Verrou, K. M., et al. (2023). SARS-CoV-2 mRNA dual immunization induces innate transcriptional signatures, establishes T-Cell memory and coordinates the recall response. *Vaccines (Basel)*, 11(1):103.

Sandborn, W.J., Nguyen, D. D., Beattie, D. T., et al. (2020). Development of Gut-Selective Pan-Janus Kinase Inhibitor TD-1473 for Ulcerative Colitis: A translational medicine programme. *J Crohns Colitis*. 14(9):1202-1213.

Sheldon, E. (2011). Rhetorical differences in RA introductions written by English L1 and L2 and Castilian Spanish L1 writers. *Journal of English for Academic Purposes*, 10(4), 238-251.

Skorupskaite, K., George, J. T., Veldhuis, J. D., et al. (2020). Kisspeptin and neurokinin B interactions in modulating gonadotropin secretion in women with polycystic ovary syndrome. *Hum Reprod*. 35(6):1421-1431.

Stea, E. D., Skerka, C., Accetturo, M., et al. (2022). Case report: Novel FHR2 variants in atypical Hemolytic Uremic Syndrome: A case study of a translational medicine approach in renal transplantation. *Front Immunol*. 13:1008294.

Swales, J. (2004). *Research genres: explorations and applications*. Cambridge: Cambridge University Press.

Swales, J., & Najjar, H. (1987). The writing of research article introductions. *Written communication*, 4(2), 175-191.

Zappen, J. P. (2019). A rhetoric for research in sciences and technologies. In *New essays in technical and scientific communication*. London: Routledge, pp.123-138.

Unit 3
Reading and Writing a Methods Section

The methods section is one of the most important aspects of a medical paper because it provides the information that the validity of the study should be ultimately judged and reports what you did and/or what you used. The main objective of this unit is to provide a clear and precise description of the experimental design and sufficient details so that the experiment could be repeated and verified by other researchers. In some medical journals, this section is called Patients and Methods, or Materials and Methods, Subjects and Methods, Controlled Trial, and Methods. Most methods sections are usually subdivided (with subheadings) into three parts: participants, measures, procedure(s). A good methods section must be written with enough information, in order to (1) enable others to repeat the experiment and assess the reproducibility of the results, and (2) allow others to judge the validity of the results and conclusions, if necessary.

Highlight

In this unit, you will

- Learn vocabulary related to translational therapeutics, clinical practice and translational medicine
- Organize move-steps from readings into writings that reflect the genre analysis of the methods section
- Recognize how surveys, cohort and case-control studies are integrated into the text
- Learn about building an academic vocabulary bank concerning the methods section
- Build a model of methods section
- Write a short cohort and case-control essay
- Write an extended methods section

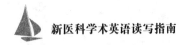

Gearing up

The following text summarizes the basic research concepts of the methods section, which is related to the principles of medical research intimately.

The scientific method attempts to discover cause-and-effect relationships between objects (ie, physical matter or processes). In the physical sciences objects are regarded as variables, and a variable is anything that can assume different values. Elucidating a cause-and-effect relationship between objects requires that variables are classified as independent, dependent, or confounding. An independent variable is one that, when manipulated, causes a change in another variable. The variable that changes in response to that manipulation is referred to as a dependent variable. For example, arterial oxygen tension is a dependent variable that responds to manipulations in independent variables such as barometric pressure and oxygen concentration. A confounding or extraneous variable is anything other than the independent variable of interest that may affect the dependent variable. Therefore, a change in a dependent variable may be due wholly or in part to a change in a confounding variable. For example, a change in minute ventilation can alter arterial oxygen tension by its effect upon alveolar carbon dioxide partial pressure.

Evaluation of a potential cause-effect relationship between two objects is accomplished through the development of the study design. A study design is simply a strategy to control and manipulate variables that provide an answer to the research question regarding potential cause-and-effect relationships.

Validity refers to the credibility of experimental results and the degree to which the results can be applied to the general population of interest. Internal validity refers to the credibility of a study and is determined by the degree to which conclusions drawn from an experiment correctly describe what actually transpired during the study. External validity refers to whether (and to what degree) the results of a study can be generalized to a larger population. Unfortunately, all biological systems are profoundly complex, so simple, unambiguous, direct relationships between objects can be difficult to ascertain. The internal validity of a study is judged by the degree to which its outcomes can be attributed to manipulation of independent variables and not to the effects of confounding variables. Therefore, the study protocol must be designed to control (eg, to keep constant) as many extraneous factors as possible so that any potential cause-and-effect relationship between two objects can be judged accurately. It is important to emphasize that confounding variables can never be fully controlled. Furthermore, the influence of these variables may not be fully appreciated by those conducting the research. External validity is primarily determined by how subjects are selected to participate in a study and by the use of randomization procedures that limit potential bias in how subjects are assigned to treatment groups.

From Respiratory Care, *2004*, *49(10)*, *1229 - 1232*, *written by R. H. Kallet.*

Work in a small group, and discuss the following questions.

1. What variables are mentioned in this text? What variables are needed to be measured and why?
2. What is the function of a study design?
3. What validities are mentioned in this text? What are the relationships between them?

Section 1　Reading

Task 1　Activating background knowledge

Task 1A　Discuss the following questions

1. What should be included in a methods section?
2. What does a well-written methodology provide? What differences are there between methodology and methods?
3. What do you think of participants selection?
4. How to describe data collection process in a methods section?

Look at Table 3.1 and tick your items, and then share your answers with your classmates.

Table 3.1　Questionnaire for writing a methods section in medical research

Questions	True	False
Question 1: What are the purposes of clearly explaining how a scientific study was conducted in a methods section?		
(1) To enable readers to evaluate the work performed		
(2) To provide a step-by-step tutorial for the readers		
(3) To permit others to replicate the study		
(4) To describe the experimental design and provide sufficient details about the study		
Question 2: Are the following contents and writing styles to be included in the materials and methods section?		

Continued

Questions	True	False
(1) Describing the materials used in the study		
(2) Explaining how the materials were prepared		
(3) Describing the research protocol		
(4) Explaining how measurements were made and what calculations were performed		
(5) Stating which statistical tests were done to analyze the data		
(6) The writing should be direct and precise and in the past tense		

Task 1B To help you to read academic medical text effectively, here are some descriptions in Table 3.2 that you are required to tick.

Table 3.2 Questionnaire for the structure and content of the methods section (Azevedo et al, 2011)

Structure and content	YES	NO
A possible structure in methods should include study design, selection of participants, data collection, data analysis.		
The study design is most frequently described, systematized and reported as follows: descriptive vs. analytical, comparative vs. non-comparative, factors and existence of randomization, type of randomization, participant selection under assessment, cross-sectional vs. longitudinal nature, prospective vs. retrospective.		
A clear presentation of the ethical considerations is mandatory in all animal or human studies.		
Selection of participants section should cover selection criteria, methods for selection of participants and recruitment process.		
The data collection process should include the variables measured and the methods and instruments used for their measurement.		
This data analysis should describe the descriptive statistics used, main types of variables analyzed, inferential methods used.		

Task 2 Understanding the facts and details

Reading 1 Text theme: Translational therapeutics

Task 2A Read the text, and fill in each blank with a proper form of the word in the bracket.

Phase Ⅱ Clinical and Translational Study of Everolimus±Paclitaxel as First-Line Therapy in Cisplatin-Ineligible Advanced Urothelial Carcinoma

Tomi Jun et al

Patients and Methods

Participants

1. Aadults patients (aged 18 or older) with histologically proven UC who were ineligible for cisplatin and who had not been previously treated for metastatic disease were eligible for this study. Upper tract disease and mixed histology (with a UC component) were allowed. Cisplatin ineligibility was based on one of two _____ (criterion): (1) calculated creatinine clearance (by the Cockroft-Gault formula) < 60 mL/minute, (2) Karnofsky performance status 60—70%. Patients meeting both criteria were assigned to cohort 1 while patients meeting only one criterion were assigned to cohort 2. Key exclusion criteria included active brain metastases and lack of measurable disease (per RECIST). Patients were enrolled from treatment centers within the US-based Hoosier Cancer Research Network.

Trial Oversight

2. The protocol was approved by the Institutional Review Board of each participating institution. Written informed consent was obtained from all participants prior to enrollment. The study was performed in accordance with ethical principles originating from the Declaration of Helsinki, which are consistent with ICH/Good Clinical Practice, and applicable _____ (deregulation) requirements.

Interventions

3. Patients in cohort 1 were assigned to take everolimus alone (EVE) at a dose of 10 mg by mouth daily, without interruption. Medications were dispensed on an outpatient basis on day 1 of each 28-day cycle. Patients in cohort 2 were assigned to a combination of EVP. Everolimus was prescribed at the same dose and _____ (reschedules) as for cohort 1. Paclitaxel 80 mg/m2 was given as a 1-hour intravenous infusion on days 1, 8, and 15 of each 28-day cycle.

4. Dose reductions were permitted in accordance with a schedule specified in the protocol. Paclitaxel could be reduced to 60 mg/m2 and everolimus could be reduced to a minimum of 5mg every other day. The study drugs were discontinued if further dose reductions were ____ ____ (requires) or if treatment was interrupted for greater than 4 weeks.

5. Treatment was continued until radiographic progression (by RECIST criteria), unacceptable toxicity, death, or discontinuation for any other reason. Cross-sectional

imaging was obtained every 2 _____(cycling) until disease progression.

Outcomes

6. The primary）objective was to evaluate CBR at 4 months from treatment initiation. Clinical benefit was defined as complete respondse（CR）, partial respondse（PR）, or stable disease（SD）per RECIST criteria. Secondary objectives were to evaluate the safety of EVE and EVP in this population, and to determine progression-free _____ (survivors)（PFS）and 1-year overall survival（OS）. Exploratory objectives included identifying genomic correlates of outcomes using whole-exome and transcriptome sequencing data from archived tumor samples.

Genomic Analyses

7. Formalin-fixed paraffin-embedded tumor and paired blood normal samples（N = 17）were submitted for whole-exome sequencing（WES）. Exome capture and sequencing library preparation were performed using the SureSelect Human All Exon V7, no UTR hybridization capture kit from Agilent（Santa Clara, CA）. Libraries were sequenced on an Illumina HiSeq 4000 instrument with 100-bp paired-end reads. An in-house GATK4-based pipeline（TIGRIS）was used to analyze the WES profiles. Somatic variants with a general allelic fraction（AF）or ethnic-specific AF $\geqslant 0.5\%$ in the gnomAD database were removed from analysis. Copy number variant（CNV）segmentation profiles were called using saasCNV, then fed into GISTIC 2.0^3 across the entire cohort to look for significant CNV _____（regional）. Mutational signature analysis was done via R package quadprog[4], and only samples with SNVs in exome region $\geqslant 50$ at AF $\geqslant 5\%$ were included, resulting a total of 14 samples. The signature fitting step was conducted using a reference catalog consisting of bladder cancer specific COSMIC v2 mutational signatures 1, 2, 5, 10, and 13.

8. RNA sequencing was performed on 8 of the 17 WES samples using SureSelect RNADirect（Agilent, Santa Clara, CA）. An in-house RNaseq data processing pipeline（EUPHRATES）was used to analyze the data. UCSC's hg19 genome build was used as the standard reference genome for all _____（analyzing）. Gene annotations were derived from UCSC's refGene table. Briefly, STAR（v2.6.1.d）was used for read alignment, and feature Counts（v1.4.4）was used to measure abundance of genomic features. Differential gene expression analysis was then performed using the DESeq2 package using read counts from the previous step. Gene fusion events were also screened for using open screened fusion calling tools FusionCatcher（v1.0）and FusionInspector(v2.1.0).

Statistical Considerations

9. The study included two parallel cohorts and was not designed for statistical

comparison of the cohorts. Each cohort used a separate Simon's two-stage minimax design, with one-sided α 0.05 and power 0.8. For cohort 1, the _____ (minimally) activity threshold was a 4-month CBR of $\leqslant 10\%$ while the substantial activity threshold was a CBR $\geqslant 30\%$. For cohort 2, the minimal activity threshold was a CBR $\leqslant 25\%$ while the substantial activity threshold was a CBR $\geqslant 45\%$.

10. Based on these parameters, we planned to accrue 15 evaluable patients in the first stage for cohort 1, and an additional 10 patients in the second stage. For cohort 2, we planned to enroll 17 patients in the first stage, and an additional 19 patients in the second stage. _____ (anticipant) a 10% dropout rate, the target accrual was 68 patients: 28 in cohort 1 and 40 in cohort 2. The trial opened in 2010 but was closed in 2018 due to slow accrual after having enrolled 36 patients: 7 in cohort 1 and 29 in cohort 2. All patients who received at least one dose of the trial medication were included in the final analyses for efficacy and safety.

11. Descriptive statistics were summarized using medians and ranges for continuous variables and counts and proportions for categorical variables. The primary outcome of 4-month CBR was calculated as the number of patients achieving clinical benefit at 4 months divided by the total number of patients in the cohort. 95% confidence intervals for proportions were calculated using the Clopper-Pearson exact method. Survival outcomes were estimated using the Kaplan-Meier method.

12. Statistical analyses were conducted in R _____ (statistically) software, version 4.0.0.

From the Oncologist, 2022, 27:432-452

Task 2B   Read the text closely. Decide whether these statements are TRUE (T) or FALSE (F).

1. The study was performed in accordance with ethical principles originating from the Declaration of Helsinki, which are consistent with ICH/Good Clinical Practice, and applicable regulatory requirements.   (   )

2. Patients in cohort 2 were assigned to take everolimus alone(EVE) at a dose of 10 mg by mouth daily, without interruption.   (   )

3. Treatment was continued until radiographic progression (by RECIST criteria), unacceptable toxicity, death, or discontinuation for any other reason. (   )

4. Clinical benefit was defined as complete response (CR), partial response (PR), or stable disease (SD) per RECIST criteria.   (   )

5. First objectives were to evaluate the safety of EVE and EVP in this population, and to determine progression-free survival (PFS) and 1-year overall survival (OS).   (   )

6. Descriptive statistics were summarized using medians and ranges for continuous variables and counts and proportions for categorical variables.   (   )

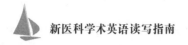

Task 3 Academic literacy skills: Reading for specific information

Task 3A Understanding facts and opinions

Opinions are personal statements in light of an individual's beliefs or attitudes. Although sometimes facts need proof, facts are recognized as impersonal statements of truths.

Discuss with your classmates and judge which of the following statements is an opinion, a fact, or a fact that needs proof. The first statement has been done for you as an example.

① Opinion   In biomedicine and related felds, people-centric research has been focusing on multiple health-related topics, ranging from quality of life (HRQoL) to information needs and symptom treatment prioritization.

② _____   The total number of items present in the ImmunoCDGQ and ImmunoHealthyQ was 58 and 56, respectively.

③ _____   Conferences and meetings were also a pursued avenue, particularly during the pre-launch and result dissemination phases (Fig. 3).

④ _____   Curative treatment options for patients with metastatic solid tumors are still rare.

⑤ _____   A high number of advanced solid tumours (30—80%) display potentially "actionable" genomic variants.

⑥ _____   reatment recommendations included a variety of FDA approved agents, including targeted oncology agents and repositioned agents.

⑦ _____   Within this feasibility study, two subjects underwent a repeat biopsy at time of progression and a second tumor board treatment recommendation was issued based on repeat WES and RNAseq.

⑧ _____   Our data confirm and improve the main results reported in the scientific literature on the importance of taking probiotics in prostatitis.

⑨ _____   Prostatitis is a prostate condition characterized by prostate inflammation, pain and a variety of urinary symptoms such as urinary frequency, urgency, dribbling and the need to urinate often at night.

⑩ _____   Research has also found that men with chronic prostatitis have lower seminal lactobacilli levels than healthy men, due to frequent antibiotic treatments.

Task 3B Moves in medical material/methodology section

In the tradition of Swalesian genre theory, move/step schemas for methods sections have been explored in Table 3.3—3.5.

Table 3.3　Biochemistry move/step schemas for methods section（Kanoksilapatham, 2005）

Move 1: Describing materials	Step 1: Listing materials
	Step 2: Detailing the source of the materials
	Step 3: Providing the background of the materials
Move 2: Describing experimental procedure	Step 1:Documenting established procedures
	Step 2: Detailing procedures
	Step 3: Providing the background of the procedure
Move 3: Detailing equipment	
Move 4: Describing statistical procedures	

Table 3.4　Psychology move/step schemas for methods section（Zhang et al, 2011）

	Step 1: Relate to prior/next experiments
	Step 2: Justify methods
	Step 3: Preview methods
	Step 4: Describe participants
	Step 5: Describe materials
	Step 6: Describe tasks
	Step 7: Outline experimental procedures
	Step 8: Present variables
	Step 9: Outline data analysis procedures
	Step 10: Present reliability/validity

Table 3.5　Inter-disciplines move/step schemas for methods section（Cotos et al, 2017）

Move 1: Contextualizing study methods	Step 1: Referencing previous works
	Step 2: Providing general information
	Step 3: Identifying methodological approach
	Step 4: Describing the setting
	Step 5: Introducing the subjects
	Step 6: Rationalizing pre-experiment decisions

Continued

	Step 1：Acquiring the data
	Step 2：Describing the data
	Step 3：Delineating experimental/study procedures
Move 2：Describing the study	Step 4：Describing tools
	Step 5：Identifying variables
	Step 6：Rationalizing experiment decisions
	Step 7：Reporting incrementals
	Step1：Preparing the data
Move 3：Establishing credibility	Step 2：Describing data analysis
	Step 3：Rationalizing data processing/analysis

Task 4　Building your vocabulary

Work with your partner，match each key word and phrase to its definition.

Word/phrase	Definition
1. criteria	**a.** place a value on；judge the worth of something.
2. sequenced	**b.** a small amount of sth that shows what the rest of it is like.
3. formula	**c.** the development of tumours in different parts of the body resulting from cancer that has started in another part of the body.
4. evaluate	**d.** ratio of the clearance function of creatinine per unit time in plasma.
5. hypothesis	**e.** serial arrangement in which things follow in logical order or a recurrent pattern.
6. categorized	**f.** the act of adding sth to sth else in order to make it stronger or more successful.
7. strategy	**g.** an instrument used in medical operations which consists of a very small camera on a long thin tube which can be put into a person's body so that the parts inside can be seen.
8. subsidiary	**h.** plural of criterion；a basis for comparison；a reference point against which other things can be evaluated.
9. interval	**i.** happening fairly often and regularly.
10. metastasis	**j.** relating to something that is added but is not essential.
11. intravenous	**k.** a system of connected organs or tissues along which materials or messages pass.

Continued

Word/phrase	Definition
12. infusion	**l.** an elaborate and systematic plan of action.
13. variant	**m.** a group of symbols that make a mathematical statement.
14. tract	**n.** a small infection lump that grows inside the body, especially in the nose, that is caused by disease but is usually harmless.
15. creatinine clearance	**o.** a definite length of time marked off by two instants.
16. endoscopy	**p.** the form and structure of animals and plants, studied as a science.
17. periodic	**q.** arranged into categories.
18. morphology	**r.** a thing that is a slightly different form or type of sth else.
19. specimens	**s.** a proposal intended to explain certain facts or observations.
20. inflammatory polyps	**t.** (of drugs or food) going into a vein.

Task 5　Understanding the text moves

Reading 2　Text theme: Clinical practice and translational medicine

Task 5A　Read the text, and fill in each blank with a proper form of the word in the bracket.

Artificial Intelligence-Assisted Optical Diagnosis for the Resect-and-Discard Strategy in Clinical Practice: The Artificial Intelligence BLI Characterization (ABC) Study

Emanuele Rondonotti et al

Centers and patients

1. This prospective cohort study was conducted in four open-access endoscopy centers in Italy (listed in Appendix 1s, see online-only Supplementary Material). The institutional review boards of all participating centers approved the protocol. All patients provided their written informed consent. The study is reported according to STROBE guidelines.

2. Consecutive adults (18-85 years) undergoing outpatient colonoscopy were considered for inclusion, with enrollment limited to those patients in whom at least one DRSP was detected. The _____ (exclude) criteria are listed in the Appendix 2 s.

Study outcomes

3. According to the Preservation and Incorporation of Valuable endoscopic innovations

(PIVI)-1 threshold, proposed by the American Society of Gastrointestinal Endoscopy, the primary end point was to assess whether AI-assisted optical diagnosis with a high degree of confidence achieved $\geq$ 90% NPV for adenomatous histology of DRSPs, having histopathology as the reference standard. The secondary aims were: (i) to calculate the performance measures of the endoscopist alone (endoscopist-alone optical diagnosis) and the AI system alone (AI-alone optical diagnosis); (ii) to evaluate whether the post-polypectomy surveillance interval based on optical diagnosis achieved $\geq$ 90% agreement (the PIVI-2 threshold) according to both the United States Multi-Society Task Force (USMSTF) and European Society of Gastrointestinal Endoscopy (ESGE) guide-lines.

4. We also planned exploratory subgroup analyses on accuracy according to the level of _____ (expert) (i. e. expert vs. nonexpert), level of confidence (i. e. high vs. low), and polyp location (i. e. rectosigmoid vs. nonrectosigmoid polyps).

Endoscopic _____ (proceed)

5. All procedures were performed using the ELUXEO 7000 endoscopy platform (EC-760ZPV and EC-760RV endoscopes, ELUXEO VP-7000 videoprocessor, and ELUXEO BL-7000 light source; Fujifilm Co.).

6. The participating endoscopists were dichotomized as experts (had followed a dedicated training program, _____ (undergo) periodic auditing and monitoring, and performed optical diagnosis on a regular basis, according to the ESGE curriculum) and nonexperts in optical diagnosis. Regardless of their expertise, all endoscopists received formal training, which consisted of a 45-minute lecture on the principles of optical diagnosis, the blue-light imaging (BLI) system, the BLI Adenomas Serrated International Classification (BASIC) system, and the features of the AI system used in the present study.

AI system

7. A real-time convolutional neural network-based AI system (CAD-EYE) was used for polyp characterization in BLI mode. The technical features of the system have been described else-where. Briefly, the AI system provides optical diagnosis through: (i) polyp _____ (identify) in the "location map"; (ii) colored brackets surrounding the endoscopic image; and (iii) diagnostic labeling as "hyperplastic" or "neoplastic" (i.e. adenoma or nonadenoma, according to the manufacturer's indication). ▶ Fig.1 shows how the CAD-EYE output is provided.

Steps involved in AI-assisted optical diagnosis

8. All polyps identified by the endoscopist had their size, location, and morphology (according to the Paris classification) reported. They were resected and retrieved in separate jars and sent for pathology _____ (assess).

9. All $\leq$ 5-mm polyps were characterized (as adenomas or nonadenomas) through a

three-step _____ (sequence) process. Every step of polyp optical diagnosis was performed with BLI and in real time during the endoscopic procedure.

10. In the first step (endoscopist-alone optical diagnosis), the endoscopist categorized the polyp as an adenoma or nonadenoma, using the BASIC classification, without AI _____ (assist). The endoscopist's confidence level in the optical diagnosis (high vs. low) was recorded. Only DRSPs evaluated with high confidence were included in the analysis of endoscopist-alone performance.

11. In the second step (AI-alone optical diagnosis), the AI system was switched on and the output that was automatically provided by the AI system (adenoma vs. nonadenoma) was recorded, irrespective of the previous output and level of confidence of the endoscopist. The AI output was collected only when the system was able to provide it and it was technically _____ (rely) and stable over time. Further details about the CAD-EYE user interface and operation are reported in Appendix 3 s.

12. In the third step (AI-assisted optical diagnosis), the final diagnosis (adenoma vs. nonadenoma) provided by the endoscopist combining the results of the first two steps was reported, as well as the confidence level (high vs. low). Only DRSPs receiving a high confidence AI-assisted optical diagnosis were used for the _____ (compute), irrespective of the results of the previous steps.

Pathology (reference standard)

13. Expert pathologists (at least one in each center), blinded to the optical diagnosis, evaluated all the resected polyps according to the Vienna classification. For the present study, hyperplastic polyps, sessile serrated lesions, inflammatory polyps, or normal mucosal samples were all labeled as nonadenomas. Taking into account the dichotomy "adenoma" and "nonadenoma," if disagreement between the pathological diagnosis and high confidence AI-assisted optical diagnosis of DRSPs was disclosed, the pathology specimens were blind lyre viewed by a second expert pathologist and the polyp was then reclassified by agreement. Adenomas with significant villous features (> 25%), size ≥ 1.0 cm, high grade _____ (dysplasia), or early invasive cancer were defined as advanced.

Statistical analysis and sample size calculation

14. With an expected prevalence of rectosigmoid adenomas of 46.8%, based on previous data collected in the centers participating in the present study, an NPV for AI-assisted diagnosis of > 90% implied a < 0.11 likelihood ratio for negative results. Using the _____ (equate) described by Simel et al., we determined the minimum sample size required to test the primary hypothesis (at 5% two-sided significance level and 80% power) to be 235 adenomatous DRSPs.

15. With regard to the post-polypectomy surveillance intervals, the optical diagnosis-based strategy was calculated taking into account high confidence optical diagnosis

of $\leqslant$ 5-mm polyps, along with the histopathological assessment of both polyps $\geqslant$ 6-mm in size and those of $\leqslant$ 5 mm that were evaluated with low confidence. If only diminutive polyps were detected and evaluated with high confidence, the optical diagnosis-based post-polypectomy surveillance intervals was provided at the end of the endoscopic procedure; otherwise, it was made as soon as the histopathology became available.

16. Comparisons of categorical variables were performed by two-sided chi-squared test or Fisher exact test, as appropriate. AP value of $\leqslant$ 0.05 was considered statistically significant for our primary outcome measure. All other outcome measures (e.g. diagnostic performance according to the level of endoscopist expertise) were treated as secondary in our study design. There was no need to adjust for multiplicity, as findings for secondary outcome were considered _____ (subsidy) and exploratory, rather than confirmatory.

From Endoscopy, 2023, 55(1): 14-22

Task 5B Read the text carefully and decide what the moves are.
1. Why do the authors describe the experimental subjects first?
2. How do the authors describe the experimental procedures?
3. What are the functions of endoscopic procedures and AI system?
4. What's the major experimental procedure?
5. How do the authors deal with the statistics?

Section 2 Writing

Task 6 Warm-up writing assignment

Task 6A Grammar and phraseology in a medical methods section

1. Tense and voice in a medical methods section

The methods section should be written in simple English, in the past tense, active voice or passive voice and tense pairs. The procedure used in the mtethods section is described in the passive, either in the present simple passive or in the past simple passive.

(1) The passive is used when the writer wants to focus on the result, not on the cause

> ① The Medline database PubMed and Google Scholar **were selected** to retrieve both indexed and grey literature.
> ② A 24-year-old Caucasian man **was referred to** the nephrology unit for a pre-transplantation kidney evaluation.

③ Eighteen SARS-CoV-2-naïve healthy healthcare professionals 28—65 years old **were enrolled** in the study between January and December 2021 under informed consent.

④ Wild type C57BL/6J and B6. C（Cg）-Cd79atm1（cre）Reth/EhobJ （"Cd79aCre/＋", also known as Mb1-Cre49）mice **were obtained** from The Jackson Laboratory.

①—④ use the past simple tense to describe what you did.

⑤ Description of its scientific content development, piloting, translation, and ethical submission **are reported in and detailed in** the checklist for reporting results of internet E-Surveys.

⑥ The immunization schedule and sample collection time-points **are illustrated** in Figure 1.

⑦ Once the regulons are constructed, the method AUCell scores individual cells by assessing for each TF separately whether target genes **are enriched** in the top quantile of the cell signature.

⑧ First TF-gene co-expression modules **are defined** in a data-driven manner with GRNBoost2.

⑨ To improve compliance, the simplicity and saliency of "repetitive swallowing" over the more demanding and complicated exercises **is investigated** in the current study.

⑤—⑨ use the present simple tense to describe what is normally done or to describe a standard piece of equipment used in the research.

(2) In most methods sections, the active and the passive are mixed, written in the past tense preferably. Read the following text and underline the passives.

Eighteen SARS-CoV-2-naïve healthy healthcare professionals 28—65 years old were enrolled in the study between January and December 2021 under informed consent. Prior to enrollment, previous COVID-19 infection was excluded using an in-house-developed ELISA. Subjects with major comorbidities（malignancies, immunosuppression, chronic kidney disease, liver failure, genetic syndromes）were excluded. All participants received two primary doses of the Pfizer-BioNTech mRNA BNT162b2 vaccine 3 weeks apart followed by a third dose 10 months later. Whole blood samples for peripheral blood mononuclear cell（PBMC）isolation were collected prior to the second dose（Day 21, D21）and three weeks after the second dose（Day 42, D42）; samples for transcriptome analysis were collected on D21 and three days after the second dose（Day

24，D24）；sera for RBD-specific antibody enumeration were collected on Days 21 and 42 and 3 weeks after the third dose（Month 11）. The immunization schedule and sample collection time-points are illustrated in Figure 1.

　　……

Continuous variables are presented as mean or median values. All comparative statistical analyses were performed using either a two-sided t test when the variable was normally distributed，or a nonparametric test if not. Relationships were assessed using mono-or multi-variant analysis methods. Statistical significance was set at $p = 0.05$ and analyses were conducted using GraphPad（v6）.

2. Phraseology in medical methods sections

（1）Describe previously used methods

Clinical application of dPCR in viral DNA quantification several studies **have utilized** dPCR to directly quantify DNA viremia loads in clinical samples.

A critical appraisal using a specific **tool** was conducted to **assess** the quality of each included study.

Traditionally，hyperandrogenemia has **been assessed by measuring** total-testosterone.

Various **methods have been proposed to** analyze a weighted summary proportion.

We have examined the diagnostic value of preoperative and intraoperative **non-invasive methods** to **determine** the lymph node status...

ECEs' physical activity and sedentary behavior-related self-efficacy has been **measured** in a **variety** of **ways** in childcare-based research.

This method has been successfully **used in** clinical and experimental studies and results in localization precision that is comparable with...

Two main theories have **attempted** to **account** for cross-domain interactions.

Linear regression was **utilized to assess** correlation of continuous variables.

In this work，we **propose** a computational tool to **quantify** pluripotency from single cell transcriptomics data.

Herein，the authors **proposed** to assess the viability of **measuring** the TMM speed of sound in the water/glycerol maintenance solution.

To overcome this shortcoming，we **propose** a new motion model that **captures** the motion field on...

（2）Give reasons why a particular method was adopted

A **major advantage** of a meta-analysis is that it produces a precise estimate of the effect size, with considerably increased statistical power...

A mixed model analytic **approach was used to** compare patient outcomes between the younger and elderly groups.

The SR **method** is **particularly useful** in cases where missingness occurs simultaneously for multiple participants, such as concurrent...

A qualitative and **quantitative approach** was adopted divided into six steps...

We suggest several **practical ways** to enhance the uptake of open science principles...

Polymer optical fiber （POF） sensors have **attractive features** for smart textile technology, and combined with Artificial Intelligence...

DNA vaccines have the **advantage** of being **simple** to construct, produce and **deliver**.

We concentrate on four **case studies** to **offer** a theoretically-grounded analysis which attends to the relationship between.

While this study has the **advantage of using** a geographically and institutionally broad data source, our conclusions may not be generalizable to...

The **advantage of using** AF for CMV quantitative PCR is that it can be done on the fluid sampled and used to establish prenatal diagnosis.

（3）Describe the characteristics of the sample

The overall **population** was **divided** into **two groups according** to female age: the Vienna consensus （39 years） and older female age （40 years）.

A **random sample** of GHS participants （$n = 59$） was **recruited** to take part in semistructured interviews about their perceptions and experience...

This cohort **study** aims to **recruit** around 5000 Swedish full-time **students**.

Students were **recruited** from six schools. **Students** participated in a standard CPR training program provided by tutors.

The **sample** consisted of 225 students, out of which 113 were males and 112 were **females**.

Three **samples** of young Arab **females** were chosen from different young **female** populations （$n = 450$）.

We extracted **selection criteria** from the transcripts of the audio-recorded interviews and **identified** other factors that influenced selection.

Seventy-two **participants** were **divided** equally into 3 groups: proprioceptive training with...

Subjects were **interviewed** at baseline in person, answered **interview** questions at 6 months via computer...

Eleven pairs of **subjects** were **interviewed** twice using 24-hour dietary recalls such that each member of the pair...

Semi-structured interviews were conducted among 40 **participants** (19 male and 21 female) **aged** between 67 and 92 years...

Sixteen general practitioners (GPs) were **recruited** to **participate** in one-to-one interviews, eighty health and social care professionals working in...

(4) Describe the process of the experiment

Before conducting statistical analyses, the volumes of each subcortical region of interest **were normalised** for head size via multiplication by...

The **ethical approval was obtained** from the Western Institutional Review Board, George Washington University IRB, JPS Health Network IRB...

Drugs were administered over several 3 days on/3 days off cycles initiated when the tumors first became palpable...

These **data were generated** over five assays conducted during a 1-week period.

In this study, the unaffected ears **were used as** a normal standard for signal intensity ratio calculation...

Data were **collected** through **semi-structured interviews**, between April and October 2015, and analyzed by the constant comparison method.

Blood **samples were taken from** the antecubital vein to 3.8% sodium citrate in a proportion of 9:1 (v/v).

Selection of Participants **Data were gathered from** September 2012 through January 2013.

All **the experiments were conducted** according to the National Institutes of Health Guide for the Care and Use of Laboratory Animals.

In this multiphase multicenter study, peripheral **blood samples were obtained** preoperatively in 3 phases...

Independent evaluation of six genomic **tests** was **carried** out by a panel of experts in three parameters...

At 10-minute increments, **the participants were asked to** answer 7 questions (with provided answer choices)...

During this control period, all **the participants were asked to** continue their regular lifestyle and refrain from making changes to their diet.

Task 6B Literacy skills: Surveys, cohort and case-control studies

1. Surveys

Surveys, are used most usually to describe a method of gathering information from a sample of individuals and provide a crucial source of basic scientific knowledge. Surveys can be classified into three main types: self-completed, interviewer-assisted or completed (Scheuren, 2004).

(1) The type of survey

① Postal survey

A survey's design is one in which an unsolicited questionnaire arrives either through the post, or in email, which objectives should be as specific, clear-cut, and unambiguous as possible.

Postal survey—Healthy Mothers Healthy Families Survey

The 2008 Healthy Mothers Healthy Families Survey, a **postal survey** of women 6 months postpartum in Victoria and South Australia, showed that women with xA1xAEsocial health issues xA1xAF, such as not having enough money to buy food, serious family conflict or homelessness, were twice as likely to perceive discrimination in their perinatal care.

② Interview survey

In-person interviews are generally more expensive than those made by mail or by telephone. This is mainly owing to the costs of training and paying interviewers and of their travel costs. The costs will also increase with the complexity of the questionnaire and the amount of data analysis to be collected.

Interview survey—National Health and Nutrition Examination Survey (NHANES)

We then summed the difference between the number of expected and observed deaths in each age group and calendar year for men and women separately. Risk Factors and Screening Data Data on behavioral risk factors (cigarette smoking, obesity, and physical inactivity) and receipt of cancer screening were obtained from two national surveys: the National Health **Interview Survey**(NHIS) 20 and the National Health and Nutrition Examination Survey (NHANES).

③ Clinical examination

Clinical examination is a systematic guide to physical diagnosis. It studies the prevalence of a particular disease and attempting to find associated factors of the etiology.

Clinical examination—Clinical evaluation and outcomes

A standard **clinical examination** was performed consisting of medical history interview, physical examination (cardiovascular and respiratory systems, abdominal, neurological and rheumatological examinations) and biochemistry and hematology tests.

④ Stratification

Stratification is likely to be either proportionate or disproportionate. The purpose of stratification is to get more homogeneous responses from inside the strata.

Stratified sampling—hospital characteristics

The database is built using **stratified sampling** based on the following hospital characteristics: geographic region, trauma center designation, urban or rural location, teaching status, and hospital ownership or control.

The purpose of the stratification is to produce a nationally representative sample of U.S. hospital-based EDs.

2. Cohort studies

Cohort studies structure an available study design to evaluate associations between multiple exposures and multiple outcomes on the different sides. A key characteristic of a cohort study is that the same subjects are identified and observed longitudinally in time.

Cohort study—stroke trials

In an international, multicentre **cohort study** of 4,707 patients undergoing coronary artery bypass surgery, a one point increase in NIHSS score predicted fatal and non-fatal stroke, transient ischaemic attack and coma at hospital discharge with a specificity of 86% and sensitivity of 84%.

（1）Prospective cohort study

A prospective cohort study is a study in which exposure is assessed at baseline and the researcher follows the subjects in time to study the development of disease or mortality（Euser et al, 2009）.

> Prospective cohort study—population participants
>
> Study population participants were part of the Health ABC Study, a **prospective cohort** study of 3075 community-dwelling man and women of black and white ethnicities living in Memphis, TN, or Pittsburgh, PA, and aged 70 to 79 years at recruitment in 1996 to 1997（Rooks et al., 2002）. To identify potential participants, a random sample of white and all black Medicare-eligible elders, within designated zip code areas, were contacted.

（2）Retrospective cohort

A retrospective cohort study is a very time-efficient and quick way of completing new questions with existing data（Euser, et al., 2009）.

> Retrospective cohort study—patients
>
> There was no overlap between the cohorts in study A and B. Study A—a **retrospective study** of 273 patients investigated in the Danish Anaesthesia Allergy Centre（DAAC）during 2004-11 due to a suspected perioperative allergic reaction. Of these, 153（56%）had been exposed to propofol.

3. Case-control studies

Case-control studies can usually be restricted to designs in which one is trying to identify the risks of having become a case, and harvest important scientific findings with relatively little time, money, and effort compared with other study designs（Schulz & Grimes, 2002）.

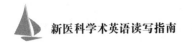

> Case-control studies—perineal laceration
>
> This was a nested **case control study** within a retrospective cohort of consecutive term vaginal deliveries at 1 tertiary care facility from 2004—2008. Cases were patients with any perineal laceration that had been sustained during vaginal delivery. Control subjects had no lacerations of any severity.

The relative advantages and disadvantages of a case-control study and cohort studies are summarized in Table 3.6.

Table 3.6　Advantages and disadvantages of a case-control, a prospective cohort and a retrospective cohort study(Machin & Campbell, 2005)

	Advantages	Disadvantages
Case-control study	• Cheap • No estimates of absolute risk • Relatively small • Only approximate estimates of relative risk • Results available quickly	• Potential biases, such as recall bias
Prospective cohort study	• Estimates of relative and absolute risk • Large and expensive • Less susceptible to bias than a case-control study	• Potential biases, such as selection bias and healthy worker effect • Results available slowly
Retrospective cohort study	• Estimates of relative and absolute risk • Results available quite quickly	• Prognostic factors limited to what has been measured in the past

Task 6C　Clinical trials

A clinical trial is defined as "a prospective study comparing the effects and value of intervention(s) against a control in human beings". It is prospective, rather than retrospective (Friedman et al, 2015).

1. Clinical trials phases

Classically, trials of pharmacokinetic studies have been divided into Phase Ⅰ, Phase Ⅱ and Phase Ⅲ.

（1）Phase I Studies

A Phase I clinical trial embarks on patients. Generally, Phase I studies attempt to assess tolerability and characteristics of the pharmacokinetics and pharmacodynamics.

Phase I trial—Myostatin antibody

Myostatin antibody significantly attenuated the muscle atrophy and loss of functional capacity in mice models of disuse atrophy. A recently conducted **phase I trial** of a myostatin inhibitor in postmenopausal women proved to increase muscle mass even in these healthy subjects, with the drug seeming to be safe and well tolerated.

(2) Phase II Studies

Once a dose or range of doses is recommended from a Phase I study, the next objective is to assess whether the drug has any biological activity or effect. Participants based on narrow inclusion criteria are typically selected in phase II studies.

Phase II trial—Intensity-modulated radiotherapy

In the Radiation Therapy Oncology Group (RTOG) 0225 study, a **phase II trial** examining the feasibility of IMRT with or without chemotherapy for NPC (stage I to stage IVB) revealed estimated 2-year locoregional progression-free and OS rates of 89.3% and 80.2%, respectively. Only 13.5% of patients had grade 2 xerostomia at 1 year. Late grade 3 xerostomia was only 3.1%, and none had grade 4 xerostomia. In Taiwan, NPC is more frequent in men than in women, with an incidence rate of 74.9% and 25.1%, respectively.

(3) Phase III Trials

① Randomized

Phase III trials are generally designed to compare the effectiveness of new interventions or existing interventions with the standard treatment for the disease in question. It is necessary to identify randomization and a random sample used in.

Randomized—Localized prostate cancer

Active monitoring, radical prostatectomy, or radiotherapy for localized prostate cancer: study design and diagnostic and baseline results of the ProtecT randomised phase 3 trial J Athene Lane, Jenny L Donovan, Michael Davis, Eleanor Walsh, Daniel Dedman, Liz Down, Emma L Turner, Malcolm D Mason, Chris Metcalfe, Tim J Peters, Richard M Martin, David E Neal, Freddie C Hamdy, for the ProtecT study group.

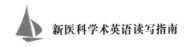

Summary Background: Prostate cancer is a major public health problem with considerable uncertainties about the effectiveness of population screening and treatment options.

② Non-randomized

Non-randomized comparative studies do not use the "gold standard" required in the randomized controlled trial. Its information is categorized as rendering poorer evidence than that from randomized trials.

Non-randomized—Recurrent stroke

Our results have implications for acute treatment after TIA and minor stroke.

First, they confirm findings from previous **non-randomized** studies for the impact of urgent treatment on the early risk of recurrent stroke, supporting recommendations for urgent assessment of patients.

Second, they suggest that most of the benefit of urgent treatment in these previous multi-intervention studies was simply due to aspirin.

Therefore, it is essential that patients with TIA or minor stroke are not sent home from the emergency department with advice to add aspirin to their next prescription; they should be treated acutely.

Similarly, patients who telephone their family doctor or advice lines should be told to take aspirin immediately.

2. Randomization

The randomized controlled clinical trial, which subjects may be selected from a larger pool of available individuals randomly, is the criteria by which all trials are judged. Randomization is a process by which each participant is likely to be assigned to either intervention or control comparably (Friedman et al, 2015). Randomization in clinical trials is of crucial importance because of bias reduction and the validity of statistical data analysis.

(1) Fixed allocation randomization

Fixed allocation randomizations in clinical trials could be prefixed proportion, adopted to allocate the entering participants among the challenging treatments. The interventions assigned to patients are prespecified probability, general equality, and that allocation probability is not variated as the study procedure. The simple, blocked, and stratified randomizations will be introduced separately in Figure 3.1.

Randomization procedures					
A. Simple randomization					

A. Simple randomization

1 Random numbers	0 7 9 4 0 3 8 7 7 0 2 9 8 0 8 5 1 7 0 8 6 4 0 8
2 Treatments (A:0—4; B:5—9)	A B B A A A B B B A A B B A B B A B A B B B A A B
3 Chronological patient N.	1 2 3 4 5 6 7 8 9 10 11 12 13 14 15 16 17 18 19 20 21 22 23 24

B. Blocked randomization

1 Random mumbers	4	1	3	6	2	6
2 Treatments	B B A A	A B A B	A A B B	B A B A	A B B A	B A B A
3 Chronological patient N.	1 2 3 4	5 6 7 8	9 10 11 12	13 14 15 16	17 18 19 20	21 22 23 24

C. Stratified randomization

1 Random numbers; stratum male	6	5	2
2 Male blocks	B A B A	B A A B	A B B A

3 Random numbers, stratum female	3	2	4
4 Female blocks	A A B B	A B B A	B B A A

5 Chronological patient N.	1 2 3 4 5 6 7 8 9 10 11 12 13 14 15 16 17 18 19 20 21 22 23 24
6 Gender of patients	M F F M F M M M F F F F M M F M M F F M M M F F
7 Treatments of males	B A B A B A A B A B B A
8 Treatments of females	A A B B A B B A B B A A

In the above table, examples of randomization methods are reported. Random numbers are obtained by "Randbetween" worksheet function provided in Microsoft Excel 2003.

A. Simple randomization. The randomization list (Row 2) is generated pairing the table of random numbers (Row 1) to the two treatments (A and B) such that A corresponds to numbers 0 to 4 and B corresponds to numbers 5 to 9. Patients (Row 3) are progressively assigned according to the obtained list.

B. Blocked randomization. The table of random numbers (Row 1) defines the entry order of the blocks. Blocks are defined through the method of "permutations with repetition." The randomization list (Row 2) is defined from: a) the entry order of blocks; b) the sequence of treatments within each block. Patients (Row 3) are progressively assigned according to the obtained list.

C. Stratified randomization. Blocked randomization is applied separately to the two strata: males and females. Patients will be assigned to the treatments following two differents lists of randomization (Row 7 for males; Row 8 for females).

Figure 3. 1   Examples of randomization methods: simple randomization, blocked randomization, and stratified randomization (Randelli et al, 2008).

① Simple randomization

Simple randomization (or complete randomization) minimizes any preferences by eradicating predictability and is adequate for large trials. The probability determined initially and the subjects allocated are in consistent with the ratio between the groups.

Simple randomization—Surgery

A minimum sample size of 30 (15 per group) was determined statistically, see below). The patients were randomly assigned into 2 groups based on computer-generated **simple randomization** of either group M (maxillary block) or group S (scalp block). Patients were premedicated with Figure 1 alprazolam 0.5 mg and ranitidine 150 mg orally on the night before and morning of the surgery.

② Blocked randomization

Blocked randomization (or permuted block randomization) is a method that can balance equal numbers of patients in sample allocation. It consists of randomizing to assign potential patients into several groups or blocks of identical size and the treatments equally (Randelli et al, 2008; Burger et al, 2021).(See Figure 3.2)

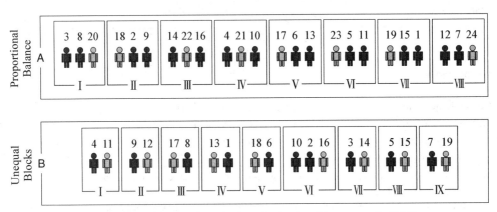

Figure 3.2　Examples of blocked randomization (Burger et al, 2021)

③ Stratified randomization

Stratified randomization is an approach which requires that the prognostic factors are examined either before or at the moment of randomization. It can reduce imbalance and increase statistical power and minimize selection bias. Although stratified randomization is well illustrated in assessing the best treatment of initial shoulder dislocation, it is not the complete solution to all potential problems of baseline imbalance. Another approach for small studies with many prognostic factors is introduced below in the section on adaptive randomization (Friedman et al, 2015).

Stratified randomization—Muscle contraction

Stratified Randomization: Prior research has shown that pain (18), sex (15), and fitness levels (22) have the potential to significantly affect muscle contraction amplitude and coordination. To control these variable, **stratified randomization** was used to allocate participants into warm-up groups. Sealed, randomly ordered opaque envelopes containing warm-up group allocations were prepared by a person not associated with the study for each of the eight subject categories detailed in Figure 2.

(2) Adaptive randomization procedures

Adaptive randomization is an important clinical trial method of changing the allocation probability based on the progress and position of the study. It may be used to minimize the imbalance between treatment groups as well as to alter the allocation probability according to the therapeutic effect. The experimental design in adaptive randomization aims to randomize the participants, allocation or proportions subjects assigned to each treatment (Rosenberger et al, 2012).

① Minimization

Minimization is a covariate adaptive randomization method to balance the prognostic factors. It provides unbiased evaluation of treatment effect and slightly increased power involved in stratified randomization (Friedman et al, 2015).

Minimization—Oncologic control

However, LPN may be a technically challenging procedure that requires considerable skill and expertise combined with the necessity to minimize ischaemic times. RPN may overcome the technical challenges of LPN. Whatever the surgical approach selected, the surgical and oncologic principles remain the same: oncologic control, preservation of renal function, and **minimization** of morbidity.

② Response-adaptive randomization

Response-adaptive randomization is "a randomization procedure that uses past treatment assignments and patient responses to select the probability of future treatment assignments, with the objective to maximize power and minimize expected treatment failures" (Rosenberger et al, 2012).

Response-adaptive randomization—Control allocation

We perform a simulation study to investigate multiple control allocation schemes within **response-adaptive randomization**, comparing the designs on metrics such as power, arm selection, mean square error, and the treatment of patients within the trial.

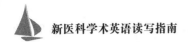

Task 7　Writing task：Build a model

Task 7A　Common models and vocabulary in medical methods sections

1. Common models of writing medical methods

Several models of scientific writing methods have been reviewed in Task 3. The model structure of information in all sections of the medical research paper was investigated using Swales'（1981，1990）genre-analysis model. Nwogu（1997）modified all moves in methods of medical research paper as follows.

Methods	Move 1：Describing data-collection procedure	Step 1：Indicating source of data
		Step 2：Indicating data size
		Step 3：Indicating criteria for data collection
	Move 2：Describing experimental procedures	Step 1：Identification of main research apparatus
		Step 2：Recounting experimental process
		Step 3：Indicating criteria for success
	Move 3：Describing data-analysis procedures	Step 1：Defining terminologies
		Step 2：Indicating process of data classification
		Step 3：Identifying analytical instrument/procedure
		Step 4：Indicating modification to instrument/procedure

Move 1　Describing data-collection procedure

Step 1：Indicating source of data

- Participating **sites in this feasibility study** included the University of California, San Francisco，(San Francisco, CA)；Children's National Health System (Washington, DC)；and the University of California, San Diego (San Diego, CA).
- Twenty-five patients with Alzheimer's disease or mild cognitive impairment, ages 50—76, were **recruited to three clinical sites**：Walnut Creek, California；San Rafael, California；and Ashland, Oregon.

Step 2：Indicating data size

- Compared to the study by Kuningas and colleagues, our **sample size** is smaller, and our power to detect CNVs with lower effect sizes is therefore reduced.

- Electronic databases were searched (MEDLINE，EMBASE，CINAHL，AMED) up to July 2015 to identify studies with objective or subjective measures of SB，**sample size** greater than 50，mean age greater than 60years and accelerometer wear time 3 days.
- Finally，the relatively small **sample size** of each study as well as the limited number of eligible studies would also affect the statistical power of our results.
- To be able to detect a difference of 20 cm h1in the area under the curve of the VAS score during coughing with an expected standard deviation of 50 cm h1，andmiu-andmiu-errors of 0.05 (two-sided hypothesis) at a power of 0.8，the calculated **sample size** was 60 patients.

Step 3：Indicating criteria for data collection

- We leveraged a two stage-procedure，whereby we intentionally chose "soft" statistical **criteria for** primary hits with a false discovery rate (FDR) of 0.66.
- The **criteria for** inclusion in the study were age greater than 18 years，ASA physical status Ⅰ to Ⅲ，and scheduled thyroid surgery.
- The inclusion **criteria for** the study were non-traumatic cardiac arrest，in patients between the age of 18 and 85 years，and the presence of endotracheal tube.
- Patient inclusion and exclusion **criteria for** this retrospective cohort study，the institutional ethics review board approved the data collection and analysis and waived the requirement for informed consent.

Move 2 Describing experimental procedures

Step 1：Identification of main research apparatus

- The cranial window was cleaned with ddH2O，and the mouse was secured under the microscope by fitting the titanium ring in a custom-built head fixation **apparatus** connected to a motorized XY stage.
- Stimulation was stopped when the reading on the plantar test **apparatus** reached 60 seconds，regardless of whether the rat showed any response.

- Stimulation was stopped when the reading on the plantar test **apparatus** reached 60 seconds，regardless of whether the rat showed any response.
- The **apparatus** was designed for contractions to be performed in the transverse plane to eliminate fatigue from lifting and lowering the mass of the forearm.

Step 2：Recounting experimental process

- Arterial pressure **was measured** using a calibrated manual sphygmomanometer，recording diastolic pressure at the 5th Korotkoff sound.
- Standard physical and neurological examinations **were performed** on each patient.
- Participants **were allowed to** consume 450 g/day（～16 ff. oz./day）caffeinated black coffee or unsweetened black tea if used to consuming them regularly.
- Animals Experiments **were conducted** on male Wistar rats aged 6 and 21 months.
- Human brain tissue Human histologically normal brain obtained from informed patients **was obtained** from the tissue depository of the Department of Neurological Surgery at the University of Washington.
- Blood samples were allowed to stand for 30—40 min，and serum separated **after** 20 min centrifugation was aliquot and stored at $-80\,^{\circ}\text{C}$.

Step 3：Indicating criteria for success

- The sample size of 100 patients provided reasonable precision for estimates of agreement with other measures of treatment success，and specific hypotheses and **criteria for success** were specified prior to data analysis.
- The **criteria for success** were based on a Cochrane review published in 2012 on the use of botulinum toxin in strabismus.
- A priori **criteria for success** of feasibility included all of the following：a response rate to the study approach letter of $=25\%$，a recruitment rate of $=80\%$ of eligible individuals，and an attrition rate at posttreatment of less than and equal to 20% and at follow-up another less than and equal to 15%.

Move 3   Describing data-analysis procedures

Step 1: Defining terminologies

- We believe that a meta-analysis of all four studies with uniform **definitions** of hormone receptor and pathological complete response is needed to identify a subgroup of patients in whom bevacizumab increases pathological complete response.
- To correct for incomparability of **definitions** of diabetes, we used regressions that converted prevalence from these sources to our primary outcome.
- Lesions **were classified** as benign if they were regular and had smooth margins, or malignant if they had irregular shape or margins.
- Abnormal lymphocytes **were classified** according to the guideline of Japanese Association of Medical Technologists.

Step 2: Indicating process of data classification

- Statistical analysis **data were collected using** Microsoft Excel and subsequent statistical analysis was carried out using SPSS release 17.0 for Windows and P less than 0.05 was considered statistically significant.
- As health-related quality of life **data were collected using** two different tools, group data (means and standard deviations) were pooled in metaanalysis softwareb using a fixed-effect model and reported as a standardised mean difference.
- Data were analysed using the software MiniTab version 15.0, and $*P$ less than and equal to 0.05; less than and equal to 0.01 **was considered significant**.
- Moreover, the Pearson correlation method was performed to evaluate the association between the painful pressure thresholds and the entropy values. P less than 0.05 **was considered significant** in all statistical analyses.

Step 3: Identifying analytical instrument/procedure

- This **was analysed using** a Wilcoxon-Mann-Whitney rank sum test with the corresponding effect size presented as Wilcoxon-Mann-Whitney generalised odds ratio with corresponding 95% CI.

- Significant group differences in protein expression were evaluated **using analysis of variance**（ANOVA）with statistical significance set to p less than 0.05.
- If the MANOVA demonstrated a significant group effect，then post hoc analyses **using analysis of variance**（ANOVA）were conducted to examine the between-group differences on the individual EF measures.
- Associations of subject baseline characteristics with CD45 − 133 + 34 + levels were investigated **using analysis of variance**（ANOVA），linear regression or non-parametric methods as appropriate.

Step 3：Indicating modification to instrument/procedure

- In addition to a 16-week behavioral **modification** and physical activity curriculum，participants in the intervention group were provided with a specific listing of healthy foods they could purchase, for which they would be reimbursed up to $25 a week.
- The predicted mechanism of inactivation involves single electron reduction of the LSD1-bound FAD cofactor, leading to homolytic cleavage of the cyclo-propyl ring, and ultimate covalent **modification** of the FAD cofactor.
- The software collapses more than 14,000 international classification of diseases，ninth revision，clinical **modification** diagnosis codes into 18 discrete，clinically meaningful categories.
- We used a **modification** of the double-level test bolus method for determination of proper injection duration with the aim of evaluating the image quality of tailored-duration CM injection compared with that of a fixed duration.
- A **modification** of magnetic twisting cytometry called optical magnetic twisting cytometry （OMTC） allows for rapid and accurate measurements of a large number of cells.
- During the MUST trial，vitreous haze was measured using a **modification** of the SUN-endorsed National Eye Institute scale16；21 in which 0.5 + haze was omitted.

2. Vocabulary in medical methods sections

（1）Provide a general introduction and overview of the materials/methods/patients/ participants and give the source of materials/patients/participants/apparatus/

equipment used. The following are some examples.

① This study **tested** the **impact** of MFS features on clinicians' progress assessments and treatment decisions in different scenarios.

② Two reviewers performed methodological quality assessment independently using a **modified version** of the Newcastle-Ottawa Scale（NOS）for observational studies.

③ The tissue processing and data collection and analysis **were performed** blind to the age of the animals.

④ The facility with which knockout **cell lines** can be **generated**, combined with a short **generation** time，makes the DT40...

⑤ Melanopsin expression was established in **all cell lines** by immunostaining or immunoblot.

⑥ In addition to the mixed-background strain，Col1a1rrr mice on a C57BL/6J background and 129 P1/ReJ background **were generated** by backcrossing for at least 9 generations.

⑦ The JAK2 biochemical kinase assay **was carried out** in Caliper format with the predominantly activated (phosphorylated) kinase domain (amino acids 808–1132).

⑧ OPK Biotech LLC（Cambridge，MA）**acquired** the former Biopure CorporationxAlxAFs assets and resumed both the manufacture and clinical development of HBOC-201.

⑨ Data were **acquired** by 12-bit A/D converter at 120 Hz using custom-built software developed in LabVIEW（National Instruments，Austin，TX）.

⑩ All the experiments were **conducted** according to the National Institutes of Health Guide for the Care and Use of Laboratory Animals.

⑪ Immunohistochemical data were **collected** and analyzed at the North-western University Cell Imaging Facility generously supported by NCI CCSG P30 CA060553 awarded to the Robert H Lurie Comprehensive Cancer Center

（2）Supply essential background information

① The baseline EPI image（ie，used for motion correction）was then **aligned with** the native T1 image using an affine transformation，followed by an affine alignment of the native T1 image to Talairach space.

② Lower limb joint rotations were defined on the basis of the initial static trial of each participant that was **aligned with** the three-dimensional laboratory coordinate system.

③ The discovery of snake DNA in mammals also shows the interesting possibility that DNA might be **horizontally** exchanged between species.

④ However，the results with the mutant are controversial，as a second study found that a large percentage of fibers were **positioned near** Ribeye-positive...

⑤ The solubilization step Membrane proteins are naturally **embedded in** a membrane bilayer constituted of a variety of proteins and lipids comprising a complex，heterogeneous and dynamic environment.

⑥ These data clearly implied that HSP70 **located downstream of** COX-2，which might exert its effects on IL-1miu regulation via the synthesis of PGE2 and cAMP.

⑦ Elongation denotes the process of peptide elongation when each amino acid **is attached to** the next via disulfide bonds according to the nucleotide sequence within the mRNA.

⑧ Acupoint LI4 **is situated** on the dorsal surface of the hand，between the first and second metacarpal bones.

⑨ Our approach **is coupled** with miniSTR multiplex PCR as an external quality control confirming the presence of a minor DNA in the studied sample.

⑩ Similarly，the calcium channel blocker cinnarizine **is connected** to the antihistamine oxatomide through binding to HRH.

⑪ The Achilles tendon **is surrounded** by connective tissue composed of both visceral and parietal layers，known as the peritenon，in place of a tendon sheath

(3) Provide specific and precise details about materials and methods

① A quality monitoring tool was **adapted** and applied.

② To support these injections，the lumbar stabilization and injection device was **adapted** and optimized for cervical intraspinal HSSC delivery.

③ Appropriate flanking primers were **added** at either 900 nM or 45 nM for the quantification and sequencing process pathways，respectively.

④ A similar approach was **adopted** with respect to collection of potential moderators for each subgroup.

⑤ Haplogroup analyses were **adjusted** for APOEe4 allele carrier status and estimated nuclear European ancestry in secondary models.

⑥ The trials in these forest plots are **arranged** to illustrate the subgroup analysis, which identified no considerable difference between the low-intensity and moderate-intensity subgroups.

⑦ The placebo pill was **assembled** by the hospital pharmacy to ensure that the placebo and the duloxetine pills appeared to be identical.

⑧ All missing values for cognitive measures were **assumed** to be missing at random and handled using maximum likelihood.

⑨ Eight small (7 mm) infrared light emitting diodes (IREDs) were **attached** to the participantxAlxAFs face to track articulatory movements of the upper lip, lower lip, and jaw.

⑩ Lactate dehydrogenase (LDH) release from cells was **calculated** as a percentage of total LDH in each sample.

(4) Justify choices made

① **To validate** this hypothesis, A172 cells were further treated with the NF-kB inhibitor KT5720 (5mium) in the absence or presence of PGE2 or forskolin.

② **In order to determine** whether or not miR-7 was upregulated in aged fibroblasts, miR-RT followed by QPCR was used.

③ **For the sake of** clarity, those data are clustered in this order and presented, step by step, in the following sections.

④ Clinical guidelines are developed **with the intention of** informing physician judgment, and often include recommendations with various degrees of scientific confldence.

⑤ Trauma team activation charges are unique to trauma centers and are used **to compensate for** costs associated with operating a trauma program and for having a trauma team available continuously.

⑥ Next, the posterior and superior tympanic bones were drilled out **to enhance** exposure.

⑦ It is hoped that these tests will provide rapid assessment of global neurological function **to facilitate** timely diagnosis and treatment of perioperative stroke.

⑧ The protocol was appositely modified **to guarantee** a progressive enhancement of effort.

⑨ Therapeutic interventions are used to try **to minimise** the severity of symptoms in triathletes after strenuous competition, such as massage, cryotherapy and stretching.

⑩ Their implication in human longevity and age-related diseases still requires more research in order **to obtain** more consistent results.

⑪ By **removing** these intended adjustments, the comparison of price-standardized amounts provides better insight into differences in resource use between critical access and non'critical access hospitals.

⑫ Two studies convincingly showed that **providing** the host with T cells against tumors in the context of a scaffold matrix created a favorable environment...

⑬ However, in patients presenting with expiratory flow **limitation**, external PEEP will not lower the expiratory driving pressure until the level of external PEEP exceeds the level of auto-PEEP by a ratio of 50 to 75%.

(5) Relate materials/method to other studies

① Another trial stated "good" adherence, **as reported by** participants in surveys; however, actual exercise attendance was 66%.

② After all, a regional technique used for intraoperative anesthesia may have a profound impact on subsequent analgesic needs, **as suggested by** the concept of preventive analgesia.

③ To further analyze this motility difference between groups, the process movement speeds were binned. **In accordance with** the initial analysis, a shift to slower process speeds with aging was again found.

④ Details on these diagnostic approaches **can be found in** the review of Freund.

⑤ Women who are heterozygous for G6PD deficiency are genetic mosaics **as explained by** the Lyon hypothesis of the X chromosome inactivation.

⑥ They have also shown that the integrated discrimination improvement (IDI) is equal to the difference in discrimination slopes **as proposed by** Yates.

⑦ Additional analyses adjusted for history of anxiety/depression **as reported in** the baseline questionnaire and restricted analysis to those women, who reported a history of anxiety/depression.

⑧ Cumulative population doublings (CPD) were assessed **as reported previously** (Frontini et al., 2011).

⑨ Interestingly, recent studies strongly suggested that oromucosal-spray cannabinoids are also effective in pain relief, **as suggested by** subjective pain rating reduction, with mild side-effects.

⑩ Caenorhabditis elegans stress resistance assays Animals were cultured in 96-well plates under conditions **identical to** those used in the lifespan assays.

⑪ Furthermore，it still remains to be determined if the energy-dissipating capacity of white adipocytes undergoing browning is **the same as that of** typical BAT.

⑫ The receiver operating curve analysis was performed，with comparison of the area under the curve (AUC) **using the method of** DeLong et al to compare the diagnostic performance between MBFabsolute and MBFratio.

⑬ All of the included studies used **a modified version of** Fried et al.

⑭ Diagnostic Assessment' Adolescents were administered **a modified version of** the World Health Organization's (WHO) Composite International Diagnostic Interview Version 3.0 (CIDI) for DSM-IV.

(6) Indicate where problems occurred

① However，emerging data on the accumulation of genome mutation in ageing human HSCs indicate that DNA damage surveillance and protection mechanisms are **not perfect** and fail during ageing.

② The present model was **not perfect**，in that it explained only 38% of the variance in length of stay.

③ We found that both methods of tissue preparation produce comparable，but **not identical**，cytocochleograms.

④ Excluding these patients in the analysis had a **negligible** effect on the results.

⑤ Locations of synapses are **unimportant** if a cell is provably electrotonically compact，but compactness can not be assumed.

⑥ Pairwise comparisons between experimental groups and the control group (STAS) were **not significant** for either prostate-cancer specific mortality...

⑦ Considering the nature of intervention studied in the included papers，blinding of participants and therapists would be **impractical**，so scores above eight would not be anticipated.

⑧ It is also possible that power to detect genetic signals was reduced due to **unavoidable** heterogeneity in cognitive assessment methods across cohorts...

⑨ Although the systemic route of rotenone may more accurately mimic human exposure to agricultural pesticides，this PD model was **limited by** its systemic toxicity.

⑩ For the combined ventilation and perfusion DECT，the radiation dose values have been **inevitably** increased because CT scan performed twice（'531 mGy x cm）.

⑪ Participants listened to the sentences and pressed a response key to indicate whether the disambiguating word was an **acceptable** or unacceptable condition...

⑫ Overall，patients with untreated asymptomatic chondral defects did **fairly well** with modified Noyes scores of 93 to 94 at over 8-year follow-up.

Task 7B Build models and move analysis

1. Build models

（1）Content and writing style of the methods section

The writing of the methods should be clear，direct，precise and accurate. The following contents should be included（Kallet，2004）：

① Subjects：Describing the materials used in the study

② Ethical considerations and preparations：Explaining how the materials were prepared

③ Protocol design：Describing the research protocol

④ Measurements and calculations：Explaining how measurements were made and what calculations were performed

⑤ Data analysis：Stating which statistical tests were done to analyze the data

（2）Methods model in medical research articles

The model of the methods section is to illustrate the usage of materials/participants/patients and the experimental procedure in the medical research article.

Methods Model for Medical RA（Huang，2014）

Move 1：Describe study materials	1：Size of study sample	
	2：Length of study period	
	3：Type of data that was collected	
Move 2：Provide inclusion criteria	1：The criteria patients/subjects required to meet in order to participate in the study	
	2：Explanation of the collected data	
Move 3：Describe procedures	1：Randomization	
	2：Measurements taken	
	3：Outcomes	
Move 4：Present the analysis of the experiment	1：Statistical test techniques	
	2：Software used	

（3）Build a model

**A Translational Randomized Trial of Perioperative
Arginine Immunonutrition on Natural Killer Cell Function in
Colorectal Cancer Surgery Patients**
Leonard Angka, Andre B. Martel, Juliana Ng, et al.

Methods

Trial Design

1. This single-center, placebo-controlled, double-blind, randomized interventional trial was approved by the Ottawa Health Science Network Research Ethics Board (20160732 – 01H) and conducted between March 2017 and July 2019 at The Ottawa Hospital. **2**. The trial was prospectively registered at clinicaltrials.gov (NCT02987296).
3. The study enrolled 24 CRC patients, and their baseline (BL) blood collection was obtained upon their written consent. **4**. The participants then were randomized to receive the isocaloric/isonitrogenous control supplement or the AES at a one-to-one ratio and instructed to take three doses per day (TID) for 5 days before and after their scheduled surgery day (SD) (Fig. 1). **5**. The surgeries were completed by two surgical oncologists (R.C.A. and S.T.).

Participants

6. Patients were eligible for the study if they were older than 18 years and had primary CRC undergoing surgical resection (including malignant polyps), adequate kidney function (creatinine clearance [30 mL/min) and hemoglobin levels ([90 mg/dL), and capability of giving written consent. **7**. Patients were ineligible if they met any of the following exclusion criteria: recent neoadjuvant chemotherapy or radiation therapy within 8 weeks of surgery; significant immunodeficiency due to illness or medication; hypotension (resting blood pressure \90/50 mmHg); history of autoimmune disease; active infection; pregnancy or nursing; severe asthma; inherited guanidinoacetate methyltransferase deficiency (inability to convert arginine to creatine); history of liver cirrhosis, heart failure, or significant cardiac disease (myocardial infarct or life-threatening arrhythmia within the preceding 6 months); or medical or psychological illness that would preclude expected compliance with the protocol.
8. One patient in the control supplement cohort withdrew consent to participate before consuming any preoperative doses and was removed from the analysis. **9**. Another patient in the control group declined to have blood drawn at any of the postoperative time points.

Intervention, Randomization, and Blinding

10. The AES and the placebo isocaloric/isonitrogenous supplement were provided by Enhanced Medical Nutrition (EMN), and their composition can be found in Fig. S1. **11**. The AES contained 4.2 g of arginine per dose, and the participants were instructed to take three doses per day for a total amount of 12.6 g arginine per day. **12**. Randomization of the order (www.random.org) by EMN enabled either AES ($n = 12$) or control ($n = 12$) supplements to be given as participants enrolled in the study. **13**. Both the investigators and the participants were blinded to the allocation. **14**. The participants received the study intervention in unmarked packages and were instructed to record and return any unused doses. **15**. The master list was unblinded only after the completion of all correlative assays and data collection.

Objectives

16. The primary objective was to compare the reduction in NK cytotoxicity (NKC) immediately after surgery (SD1 to SD0) between the control supplement and AES cohorts. **17**. The secondary objective was to compare arginine levels at all time points and the level of pre-and postoperative compliance between the groups. **18**. Additionally, we assessed the level of NK activity (NKA) and the changes in NK and MDSC frequencies at all time points.

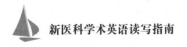

Continued

Patient Blood Processing and Storage

19. Patient and healthy volunteer blood was drawn into BD Vacutainer sodium-and heparin-coated tubes（* 40 mL/blood draw；Becton，Dickinson and Company，Franklin Lakes，NJ）. Of the whole blood，1 mL was aliquoted into Vacutainer tubes containing Promoca，30 and the remaining blood was used to isolate peripheral blood mononuclear cells（PBMCs）by Ficoll density centrifugation before cryopreservation.

Immune Assays

20. *Natural Killer Cytotoxicity（NKC）Assay*. From cryopreserved PBMCs，NKC was measured at all time points via a fluorescence-based cytotoxicity assay against K562 targets labeled with CP450 （eBioscience，San Diego，CA）. **21**. Cryopreserved PBMCs were thawed，then incubated with 0.1 mg/ mL DNAse-1（STEMCELL Technologies，Vancouver，BC）for 15 min at room temperature and finally rested overnight at 37℃ in 0.025 mg/mL of DNAse-1，10% FBS RPMI1640 media.

22. The following day，the PBMCs were washed，counted，and plated in triplicates with CP450 – K562 target cells for 4h at 37℃ at increasing effector-to-target ratios（10：1，40：1，and 80：1）.

23. Killing assay results are represented as either "NK cell cytotoxicity" quantified by percentage of dead K562 or "normalized cytotoxicity," calculated by normalization to matched patient SD0 values.

24. *Natural Killer Activity（NKA）Assay*. The ability of NK cells to secrete IFN-c in response to stimuli（NKA）was measured by enzyme-linked immunosorbent assay（ELISA；ATGen Canada/ NKMax）after overnight incubation in Vacutainer tubes containing a proprietary cytokine cocktail （NK-Vue tubes；ATGen Canada/NKMax，Montreal，QC），as previously described. **25**. Samples were given a value equal to the upper limit of detection（4000 pg/mL）or lower limit of detection（11 pg/ mL）if values fell outside the assay parameters.

26. *Flow Cytometry Profiling of Immune Cell Populations*. Freshly isolated PBMCs were used to characterize the expansion of SX-MDSCs by flow cytometry using CD33，CD11b，CD14，CD15，human lymphocyte antigen（HLA）-DR，and lineage markers（CD3，CD56，CD19）.

27. Cryopreserved PBMCs were used to characterize NK cells and monocytes using CD3，CD56，CD16（BD Horizon，Becton，Dickinson and Company Franklin Lakes，NJ），and CD14 （eBioscience）. **28**. Samples were run on either the BD Fortessa LSRII（immunophenotyping）or the BD FACsCelesta（NKC）（Becton，Dickinson and Company Franklin Lakes，NJ）and analyzed with FlowJo v10（Flowjo，Ashland，OR）.

29. *Blood Amino Acid Testing*. Fresh blood samples were collected on Whatman 903 Protein Saver Cards（SigmaAldrich，St. Louis，MI）at all time points and immediately stored at – 20℃ until batch analysis. **30**. A panel of amino acids（arginine，ornithine，citrulline，argininosuccinate，and leucine） then were measured via liquid chromatographytandem mass spectrometry（LC-MS/MS）at Newborn Screening Ontario，Children's Hospital of Eastern Ontario.

Sample Size and Statistical Analysis

31. All figures and reported values are presented as medians and interquartile ranges（IQRs）unless otherwise specified. **32**. Unpaired，non-parametric Mann-Whitney U tests were performed for comparisons between the AES and control supplement groups at any given time point，and paired Wilcoxon rank-sum tests were used to compare matched patient samples at different time points.

33. We hypothesized that a clinically relevant difference between the AES and control groups would be a 50% improvement in the degree of NK cell suppression on SD1. **34**. Based on previous ex vivo studies，the estimated reduction in NKC on SD1 was 0.54 ± 0.22 in the control cohort. A 50% improvement would be a reduction of 0.27 in the AES group. **35**. Given this baseline data，the sample size of 12 patients per group provided 80% power to detect a 50% improvement in the experimental cohort at a significance level（alpha）of 0.05.

From Annals of Surgical Oncology，2022，29（12）:7410 – 7420.

2. Move analysis: Analyze the move structures of the above model

In Sentences 1 – 2, the writers offer a general overview of the entire research design, including the location, funding, and source of data.

In Sentence 3, the writers describe baseline conditions, associated baseline measurements, and ethical considerations.

In Sentences 4 – 5, the writers describe the process of participants' recruitment, the overview of procedures executed.

In Sentence 6, the writers provide the selection of participants—selection criteria and selection methods, including the basic demographic profile of the sample population and their relevant characteristics.

In Sentence 7, the writers provide the exclusion criteria of the ineligible participants.

In Sentences 8 – 9, the writers describe all relevant aspects of clinical management not controlled by the protocol in the peri-experimental period.

In Sentences 10 – 11, the writers provide the source, type and size of the samples.

In Sentences 12 – 13, the writers provide details about what was randomized and blinded.

In Sentences 14 – 15, the writers provide details about the condition of intervention and data collection.

In Sentences 16 – 18, the writers make clear of the objectives of the procedure related either to the research question or to the entire protocol.

In Sentence 19, the writers provide the detailed process of the experiment and show the collection and reserve of materials.

In Sentences 20 – 21, the writers provide detailed information about measurements taken and also show care taken.

In Sentences 22 – 23, the writers provide detailed information about the experimental process and also describe the outcome measures.

In Sentences 24 – 25, the writers provide measurements made and experimental materials respectively and show that care was taken in detail.

In Sentences 26 – 28, the writers provide measurements made and experimental materials respectively, including identification of main research apparatus and recounting experimental process.

In Sentences 29 – 30, the writers provide measurements made and experimental materials by referring to existing methods in the literature respectively, including identification of main research apparatus, recounting experimental process and indicating criteria for success.

In Sentences 31 – 32, the writers describe more detailed information about the data-analysis procedures, including statistical test techniques and software used.

In Sentences 33 – 35, the writers further explain the statistical tests done, display

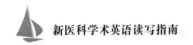

the method of analyzing the data，and shows it to have been a good choice.

3. The model rebuilt

The sentence types can reconstruct basic components of the structure methods，see the table below.

Moves	Steps
Move 1： A general introduction and contextualization of the study methods/materials	Step 1：Restate the purpose and design of the work Step 2：Give the source of materials/equipment/instrument/apparatus used Step 3：Supply essential background information，and Justify choices made Step 4：Describe the materials used in the study
Move 2：Describe specific and precise details about study materials/methods	Step 1：Size of study sample Step 2：Length of study period Step 3：Type of data that was collected Step 4：Describe the criteria patients/subjects were required to meet in order to participate in the study Step 5：Explain how the materials were prepared Step 6：Explain the data that was collected Step 7：Indicate that appropriate care was taken
Move 3：Describe experimental procedures	Step 1：Randomization Step 2：Explain how measurements were made and taken Step 3：Data collection—variables，methods，instruments and main research apparatus Step 4：What calculations were performed and outcomes Step 5：Indicate criteria for success
Move 4：Present the analysis of the experiment	Step 1：Identify the statistical tools used in the study Step 2：State which statistical tests were done to analyze the data Step 3：Describe statistical test techniques Step 4：Introduce software used

Task 8　Final assignment：Write an effective materials and methods section

Search "Translational Therapeutics" or "Clinical practice and translational medicine" on the internet，or use a sample provided by your instructor. Write an effective **materials and methods section** about translational therapeutics. Write an extended cohort and case-control study essay to describe randomization in the field.

- Revise the introductions and thesis statement, as well as your conclusion, to indicate that this essay includes more information about randomization.
- Evaluate the research performed and replicate the study, if necessary.
- Provide a clear and precise description of how the study was performed and the rationale for the methodological choices and characteristics of the study design
- Material in each section should be organized by topics from most important to least important.

Further reading

Angka, L., Martel, A. B., Ng, J., et al. (2022). A Translational Randomized Trial of Perioperative Arginine Immunonutrition on Natural Killer Cell Function in Colorectal Cancer Surgery Patients. *Ann Surg Oncol*, 29(12):7410 – 7420.

Atlantis, E., Chimoriya, R., Seifu, C. N., et al. (2022). Enablers and barriers to implementing obesity assessments in clinical practice: a rapid mixed-methods systematic review. *BMJ Open*, 12(11):e063659.

Azevedo, L. F., Canário-Almeida, F., Fonseca, J. A., Costa-Pereira, A., Winck, J. C., & Hespanhol, V. (2011). How to write a scientific paper-Writing the methods section. *Revista portuguesa de pneumologia*, 17(5), 232 – 238.

Burger, B., Vaudel, M., Barsnes, H. (2020) Importance of Block Randomization When Designing Proteomics Experiments. *J Proteome Res*. 20(1):122 – 128.

Cotos, E., Huffman, S., & Link, S. (2017). A move/step model for methods sections: Demonstrating rigour and credibility. *English for specific purposes*, *46*, 90 – 106.

Euser, A. M., Zoccali, C., Jager, K. J., et al. (2009). Cohort studies: prospective versus retrospective. *Nephron Clinical Practice*, 113(3), c214 –c217.

Friedman, L. M., Furberg, C. D., DeMets, D. L., et al. (2015). *Fundamentals of clinical trials*. springer.

Huang, D. (2014). Genre analysis of moves in medical research articles. *Stylus*, 5(1), 7 – 17.

Jun, T., Hahn, N. M., Sonpavde, G., et al. (2022). Phase Ⅱ Clinical and Translational Study of Everolimus ± Paclitaxel as First-Line Therapy in Cisplatin-Ineligible Advanced Urothelial Carcinoma. *The Oncologist*, 27(6):432 – e452.

Kallet, R. H. (2004). How to write the methods section of a research paper. *Respiratory care*, 49(10), 1229 – 1232.

Kanoksilapatham, B. (2005). Rhetorical structure of biochemistry research articles. *English for specific purposes*, 24(3), 269 – 292.

Machin, D., & Campbell, M. J. (2005). *The design of studies for medical research*.

John Wiley & Sons.

Nwogu，K. N. (1997). The medical research paper：Structure and functions. *English for specific purposes*，16(2)，119 – 138.

Patterson，R.，Schuh，M.，Bush，M. L.，et al. (2022). Expanding Clinical Trials Designs to Extend Equitable Hearing Care. *Ear Hear*. 43(1)：23S – 32S.

Pires，L.，Wilson，B. C.，Bremner，R.，et al. (2022). Translational feasibility and efficacy of nasal photodynamic disinfection of SARS-CoV-2. 12(1)：14438.

Randelli，P.，Arrigoni，P.，Lubowitz，J. H.，Cabitza P，Denti M. (2008) Randomization procedures in orthopaedic trials. *Arthroscopy*. 24(7)：834 – 8.

Rondonotti，E.，Hassan，C.，Tamanini，G.，et al. (2023). Artificial intelligence-assisted optical diagnosis for the resect-and-discard strategy in clinical practice：the Artificial intelligence BLI Characterization (ABC) study. *Endoscopy*，55(1)：14 – 22.

Rosenberger，W. F.，Sverdlov，O.，& Hu，F. (2012). Adaptive randomization for clinical trials. *Journal of biopharmaceutical statistics*，22(4)，719 – 736.

Schulz，K.F.，& Grimes，D. A. (2002). Case-control studies：research in reverse. *Lancet*，*359*(9304)，431 – 434.

Zhang，L.，Kopak，R.，Freund，L.，& Rasmussen，E. (2011). Making functional units functional：The role of rhetorical structure in use of scholarly journal articles. *International Journal of Information Management*，31(1)，21 – 29.

Zhou，Y.，Xu，J.，Hou，Y.，et al. (2022). The Alzheimer's Cell Atlas (TACA)：A single-cell molecular map for translational therapeutics accelerator in Alzheimer's disease. *Alzheimers Dement* (NY). 8(1)：e12350.

Unit 4
Reading and Writing a Results Section

The results section is generally perceived to describe the findings from the statistical analysis of the data collected to operationalize the study hypothesis, as it 1) presents the data and statistical analysis in agreement with publication manual guidelines, 2) provides an outline and highlights key findings from the data, 3) reports data related to statistical assumptions, 4) integrates the discourse of results with tables and/ or figures, 5) considers statistical analysis concerning clinical significance, 6) includes supplementary information involving in tables, figures, and other relevant data. The results section should be written in a clear, concise, and well-organized writing style and using visual aids in the reporting of the data. The results section is often short even without interpreting the data (Snyder et al, 2019; American Psychological Association, 2022; Drotar, 2009).

Highlight

In this unit, you will

- Learn vocabulary related to artificial intelligence in translational medicine and medical diagnosis
- Recognize how visual information and statistical results are integrated into texts
- Organize move-steps from readings into writings that reflect the purposes of writing results
- Learn how to display information and present statistical data
- Learn about building a medical academic vocabulary bank involved in a results section
- Build a model for a results section
- Write a short result, integrating visual information with statistical results
- Write an extended results section concerning your field

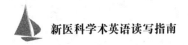

Gearing up

Work in a small group, discuss what the results section should include or avoid. Can you add any more tips or guidelines to the list?

Tips:

1. Restate hypotheses;
2. State findings;
3. State additional findings;
4. State non-validated findings;
5. Evaluate hypotheses;
6. Summarize results.

Guidelines:

1. Do not give details about irrelevant topics, such as what program was used to enter the data, while ignoring important ones (for example, which options were chosen for various statistical tests);
2. Do not report p levels of 0.0000 and negative values for t tests;
3. Do not give the p levels but not the actual values of the statistical tests;
4. Do not include confidence intervals and measures of the magnitude of an effect;
5. Do not test irrelevant hypotheses, such as whether reliability or validity coefficients are significantly different from zero;
6. Do not repeat the same data;
7. Do not write any result for a method not mentioned in "Materials and methods".

Section 1   Reading

Task 1   Activating background knowledge

Task 1A   Discuss the following questions

1. What is the goal of the results section?
2. What does the results section include?
3. What are the differences between the results section and the discussion section?
4. What descriptive statistics does the results section contain?
5. How to present the output of the analysis used to test hypotheses with a given set of data?

Look at Table 4.1, tick your items, and then share your answers with your classmates.

Table 4.1   Questionnaire for writing results section in medical research (Faryadi, 2019)

Items	True	False
① You need only to document your results scientifically.		
② When you are reporting your results, make sure they are properly organized.		
③ Report your results in the past tense as the data have already been collected.		
④ When you are declaring your results, usually use phrases such as I, We, or I found that..., we found that...		
⑤ When you are declaring your results, you may state: this research has investigated, this study has found that...and so on.		
⑥ Start from your problem statement and put forth evidence to show that you have proved or disproved the research problem.		
⑦ Interpret and discuss anything in the results section.		
⑧ Report what you have found, based on the data collected.		
⑨ Make the presentation of your results more meaningful and easier to understand.		
⑩ At the end of the results chapter, write a concluding paragraph similar to the one in the introduction.		

Task 1B   To help you to read academic medical text effectively, here are some descriptions in Table 4.2 that you are required to tick.

Table 4.2   Questionnaire for the structure and content of the results section

Structure and Content	YES	NO
① Highlight those results (including those from controls) that answer your research question.		
② Determine if the findings support or reject the hypothesis and whether they suggest clinical importance.		
③ Provide subheadings for different hypotheses or subgroup analyses.		
④ Present both descriptive values such as means, SDs, and confidence intervals as well as those from inferential tests such as the test statistic values, degrees of freedom, and significance levels.		
⑤ Give supporting information from the study using text, figures, tables, and any alternative visual aids clearly and accurately.		
⑥ Choose a presentation technique that effectively and efficiently represent the findings.		
⑦ Mention any results that contradict your hypothesis and explain why they are anomalous.		
⑧ Avoid stating outline secondary results.		

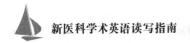

Task 2   Understanding the facts and details

Reading 1   Text theme: Artificial intelligence in medical diagnosis

Task 2A   Read the text, and fill in each blank with a proper form of the word in the bracket.

Diagnostic Accuracy of an Artificial Intelligence Online Engine in Migraine: A Multi-Center Study

Robert P. Cowan et al

Characteristics of included participants

1. A total of 266 participants were recruited to the study from the three headache centers: 143 participants from Stanford University Headache Center, 43 participants from Jan and Tom Lewis Migraine Treatment Program at Barrow Neurologic Institute, and 80 participants from George Washington University Headache Center. Of the 266 recruited participants, 202 participants completed both the CDE and SSI (study completion rate = 76%). The remaining 64 (24%) participants were excluded due to incomplete or missing data. Of the 202 participants, 102 (50.5%) were newly diagnosed (i.e., diagnosis based on SSI without a prior _____ (diagnosis) while the remaining 100 (49.5%) participants were known cases with confirmed diagnoses of different headache types. Responders had a median age of 32 years (IQR: 28, 40), female: male ratio of 3 : 1, 59% White, and 28% were recruited from headache clinics while 72% came from the local communities. The age and female: male ratio of patients recruited from the three headache centers is _____ (displaying) in Table 1. The racial demographics of participants is available in Table S2. Participants with headache had a median monthly headache day frequency of 3 (IQR = 1—13). Use of headache medication classes and frequency of monthly headache medication consumption is available in Table S3. The duration of the SSI interview as well as the time needed to complete the CDE lasted from 5 min in _____ (participated) with no headache history up to 45 min in participants reporting multiple headache types. The mean time to complete the SSI was 30 min, while the mean time to complete the CDE was 48 min.

Diagnostic accuracy performance

2. There was almost perfect concordance in M/PM diagnosis between CDE and SSI, κ = 0.82 (95% CI: 0.74—0.90; Figures 1 and 2). The CDE performed with an overall diagnostic accuracy of 91.6% (95% CI: 86.9%—95.0%), sensitivity of 89.0% (95% CI: 82.5%—93.7%), and specificity of 97.0% (95% CI: 89.5%—99.6%). postive and negative predictive values were 98.4% (95% CI: 93.9%—99.6%) and 81.0% (95%

CI: 72.5%—87.3%), respectively, using the _____ (identifies) M/PM prevalence of 67% (95% CI: 60.4%—73.7%). The age and sex ratio of SSI-based diagnosis is shown in Table 2. A 2 × 2 contingency table allowing calculations of the diagnostic performance of the CDE is displayed in Table 3. Assuming a general migraine population prevalence of 10%, the positive and negative predictive values were 76.5% (95% CI: 45.4%—92.8%) and 98.8% (95% CI: 98.0%—99.2%), respectively. The positive and negative LRs were 29.4 (95% CI: 7.5—115.1) and 0.11 (95% CI: 0.07—0.18), respectively. Based on Fagan's nomogram, a M/PM diagnosis on the CDE increases a 50% pre-test probability of having M/PM to a 97% post-test probability (Figure 2). Similarly, a negative result on CDE ("no migraine") decreases a 50% pre-test probability of having "no migraine" to a 10% post-test probability (Figure 2). If a patient from a high-risk population (i.e., headache clinic setting with a 67% M/PM prevalence) tests positive, the post-test probability that the patient truly has M/PM will be 98%. Alternatively, if the high-risk patient tests negative, the post-test probability that she or he truly has M/PM will only be 18%. For a patient from a low-risk population (e.g., _____ (communities) migraine prevalence of 10%) who tests positive on CDE, the post-test probability that the patient truly has M/PM will be 76%. On the other hand, if the low-risk patient tests negative, the post-test probability that she or he truly has M/PM will decrease to 1%. On stratified analysis, the diagnostic accuracy of CDE for M/PM diagnosis was 87%, 86%, and 82% in the subgroups of participants recruited from community, newly diagnosed participants, and known cases with confirmed diagnoses, respectively.

3. For the second analysis using "migraine" as a positive CDE and "no migraine" as a negative CDE (excluding probable migraine), there was substantial concordance in migraine diagnosis between CDE and SSI, $\kappa = 0.73$ (95% CI: 0.62—0.84). The CDE performed with an overall diagnostic accuracy of 87.2% (95% CI: 80.6%—92.3%), sensitivity of 84.0% (95% CI: 75.1%—90.8%), and specificity of 93.6% (95% CI: 82.5%—98.7%). Positive and negative predictive values were 96.3% (95% CI: 89.8%—98.8%) and 74.6% (95% CI: 64.7%—82.4%), respectively, using the _____ (identifies) migraine prevalence of 67% (95% CI: 58.2%—74.4%). Assuming a general migraine population prevalence of 10%, the positive and negative predictive values were 59.4% and 98.1%, respectively. The positive and negative LRs were 13.2 (95% CI: 4.39—39.5) and 0.17 (95% CI: 0.11—0.27), respectively. Based on Fagan's nomogram, a positive CDE increases a 50% pre-test probability of having migraine to a 92.9% post-test probability. Similarly a negatives result on CDE ("no migraine") decreases a 50% pre-test probability of having "no migraine" to a 14.5% post-test probability.

4. For the third analysis using "migraine" as a positive CDE and "no migraine/probable migraine" as a _____ (negatives) CDE, there was moderate concordance in

migraine diagnosis between CDE and SSI, κ = 0.67 (95% CI: 0.57—0.77). The CDE performed with an overall diagnostic inaccuracy of 83.2% (95% CI: 77.3%—88.1%), sensitivity of 75.6% (95% CI: 66.9%—83.0%), and specificity of 94.0% (95% CI: 86.5%—98.0%). positive and negative predictive values were 94.7% (95% CI: 88.4%—97.7%) and 72.9% (95% CI: 66.1%—78.8%), respectively, using the identified migraine prevalence of 58.9% (95% CI: 51.8%—65.8%). Assuming a general migraine population prevalence of 10%, the positive and negative predictive values were 46.3% and 96.0%, respectively. The positive and negative LRs were 12.6 (95% CI: 5.33—29.6) and 0.26 (95% CI: 0.19—0.36), respectively. Based on Fagan's nomogram, a positive CDE increases a 50% pre-test probability of having migraine to 93% post-test probability. Similarly, a negatives result on CDE ("no migraine/probable migraine") decreases a 50% pre-test probability of having "no migraine" to a 21% post-test probability.

5. The _____ (summaries) of the diagnostic accuracy results is displayed in Table 4.

6. The agreement rate between CDE and SSI (Figure 3) among nine migraine-related symptoms was 47% for photophobia, 47% for aggravation by/avoidance of routine __ _____ (physically) activity, 53% for photophobia, 65% for pulsating headache, 71% for 4—72 h headache duration, 88% for headache pain intensity, 94% for nausea and vomiting, 100% for aura, and 100% for unilateral headache, ascendingly. These agreement rates were based on the 17 participants that were either false negative or false positive in M/PM diagnosis in which the CDE performed with an overall diagnostic accuracy of 91.6% (95% CI: 86.9%—95.0%), κ = 0.82 (95% CI: 0.74—0.90).

From Headache: the Journal of Head and Face Pain, 2022, 62: 870−882

Task 2B Read the text more closely. Decide whether these statements are TRUE (T) or FALSE (F).

1. A total of 266 participants were recruited to the study from the three headache centers: 143 participants from Stanford University Headache Center, 43 participants from Jan and Tom Lewis Migraine Treatment Program at Barrow Neurologic Institute, and 80 participants from George Washington University Headache Center. (   )

2. The duration of the SSI interview as well as the time needed to complete the CDE lasted from 5 min in participants with no headache history up to 45 min in participants reporting multiple headache types. (   )

3. If a patient from a high-risk population (i.e., headache clinic setting with a 67% M/PM prevalence) tests positive, the post-test probability that the patient truly has M/PM will be 98%. (   )

4. For the first analysis using "migraine" as a positive CDE and "no migraine/

probable migraine" as a negative CDE, there was moderate concordance in migraine diagnosis between CDE and SSI, $\kappa = 0.67$ (95% CI: 0.57—0.77).

(　　)

5. The positive and negative LRs were 12.6 (95% CI: 5.33—29.6) and 0.26 (95% CI: 0.19—0.36), respectively. Based on Fagan's nomogram, a positive CDE increases a 50% pre-test probability of having migraine to 93% post-test probability.

(　　)

6. The agreement rate between CDE and SSI (Figure 3) among nine migraine-related symptoms was 47% for phonophobia, 47% for aggravation by/avoidance of routine physical activity, 80% for photophobia, 65% for pulsating headache.

(　　)

Task 3　Academic literacy skills: Read for specific information

Task 3A　Understand characteristics of medical English

Medical language is usually found to be a specialised language or a language for specific purposes. English for medical purposes refers to the teaching of English for doctors, nurses, and other personnel in the medical profession. English for new medical purposes (ENMP) provides a practical and new medical orientation of language teaching, which involves purposeful learning and the channelling of new medical materials design. New medical texts are usually considered difficult since they are written in new medical language, jargon and terminology which consist of a mixture of Latin-Greek and English derivatives (Pratt & Pacak, 1969; Maher, 1986; Halliday, 2006; Fryer, 2012).

Difficulties that are characteristic of medical English include: interlocking definitions, technical taxonomies, special expressions, lexical density, syntactic ambiguity, grammatical metaphor, semantic discontinuity.

1. Interlocking definitions

E.g. Prostatitis is a prostate condition characterized by prostate inflammation, pain and a variety of urinary symptoms such as urinary frequency, urgency, dribbling and the need to urinate often at night. This can have a bacterial origin and from the etiological point of view it appears very aggressive.

Here prostatitis, prostate, inflammation, pain, urinary symptoms, urinary frequency, urgency, dribbling are in a series of interlocking definitions. Within this set, prostatitis, prostate, inflammation, pain, urinary symptoms are mutually defining, that is, they are all used to define each other.

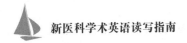

(1) Rewrite the definitions that have been mixed up in the following table.

Concept	Class	Relative pronoun or equivalent
Precision medicine	process	that tests a cancer's genetic makeup to identify molecular markers or mutations that can be targeted with treatments, has transformed cancer care and improved cancer survival
Precision cancer care	approach	which is depicted in figure 1 and described further in the following sections.
Migraines	diseases	caused by the growth of the endometrium from its normal position.
Endometriosis	disease	worldwide and a major cause of disability, with a substantial social burden

(2) Write your own definitions for the following terms.

congenital disorders of glycosylation; biobanks; atypical hemolytic-uremic syndrome; acute pancreatitis; surgical resection

2. Technical taxonomies

Medical taxonomies are not simply groups of related terms, they are highly-ordered constructions in which every term has a definite functional value.

E.g. Type species for each viral family as defined by the International Committee for **Virus Taxonomy** (ICT). Master Species List 2017 were used (ICTV2017). These included all proteins from reference viral genomes of dsRNA viruses, + ssRNA viruses and − ssRNA viruses. Protein sequences from viruses recently identified in arthropods through deep RNA sequencing studies were also included to increase the likelihood of finding sequences from divergent viruses (Cook et al, 2013; Chandler, Liu, and Bennett 2015; Li et al, 2015; Shi et al, 2016)

Medical taxonomy is typically based on two fundamental semantic relationships: type species, master species, dsRNA viruses, + ssRNA viruses and − ssRNA viruses, protein sequences, divergent viruses

(1) Discuss Figure 4.1 with your classmates, and describe the taxonomies of virus and cancer.

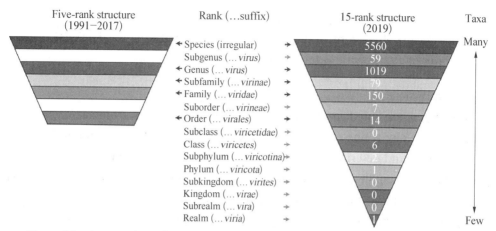

Figure 4.1 A comparison of the ICTV taxonomic rank hierarchy in 1991—2017 and 2019.

Taxonomic ranks are shown in relation to the distribution pattern of taxa. The number of taxa assigned to each rank (as recorded in the current ICTV Master Species List, release 2018b, MSL34 (ref. 47)) are shown in white font on the 15-rank structure. When the ranks are described as a hierarchy, the species rank is often referred to as the lowest rank and the realm rank as the highest rank. However, when the ranks are used as phylogenetic terms, the realm rank can be described as basal and the species rank as apical or terminal. Both conventions are used in this Consensus Statement (Salto-Tellez & Cree, 2019). See Figure 4.2.

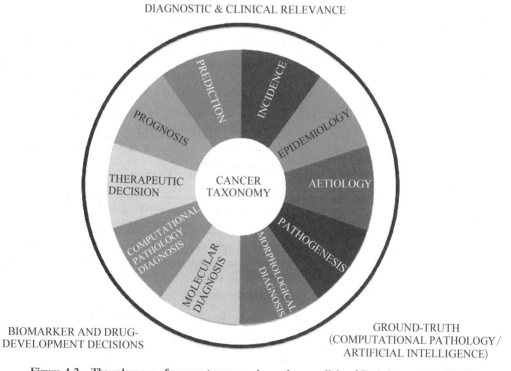

Figure 4.2 The relevance of cancer taxonomy in modern medicine (Gorbalenya et al, 2020)

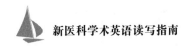

（2）Write your own taxonomies for the following terms.

breast cancer；hierarchical taxonomy of psychopathology（HiTOP）；integral taxonomy of therapeutic interventions；Parkinson's disease

3. Special expressions

Some expressions used in medical language have a special grammar of their own. Medical terminology is one of the oldest specialized terminologies in the world, which studies, analyses and describes a medical area of the lexicon. The language of medicine brings remarkable challenges to readers. Medical terms have to be named for new medicine development, for instance, terms such as endocrinology, gastroenterology, haematology, nephrology, oncology, pulmonology, rheumatology for new development of internal medicine；and the terms of computer tomography, sonograph, mammograph, laparoscope, endoscope, colonoscope, magnetic resonance image（MRI）, etc. for new diagnostic devices and methods. Main features of medical terms consist of unambiguousness, exactness, stability, word – formation potential and lack of emotionality, which bring about various relationships among them, e. g. synonymy, polysemy, hypernyms, hyponymy, etc. Its grammar can be presented in irregular plural and grammatical concord（Džuganová, 2017）. Most of English medical terms have Latin or Greek roots and are usually considered to be more difficult to learn and use for learners.

（1）Identify the polysemy of medical terminology in the following table.

Terms	Meanings
① suture	**a.** that branch of medicine which treats diseases, injuries, and deformities by manual or operative methods
	b. the place in a hospital or doctor's or dentist's office where surgery is performed.
	c. in Great Britain, a room or office where a doctor sees and treats patients
	d. the work performed by a surgeon
② surgery	**e.** the growing of plants or breeding of particular animals in order to get a particular substance or crop from them
	f. a group of cells or bacteria, especially one taken from a person or an animal and grown for medical or scientific study, or to produce food；the process of obtaining and growing these cells
	g. art, music, literature, etc., thought of as a group
	h. the beliefs and attitudes about sth that people in a particular group or organization share

Continued

③ culture	**i.** a type of fibrous joint in which the opposed surfaces are closely united, as in the skull; see sutura
	j. material used in closing a surgical or traumatic wound with stitches.
	k. a stitch or series of stitches made to secure apposition of the edges of a surgical or accidental wound; used also as a verb to indicate the application of such stitches
	l. the act or process of uniting a wound by stitches.

（2）Match Column A with Column B of synonyms in medical lexicon

Column A	Column B
1. cancer	**a.** tumour
2. erythrocyte	**b.** normocyte
3. haematopoiesis	**c.** sanguinification
4. erythrocyte	**d.** normocyte
5. cranium	**e.** skull
6. femur	**f.** thighbone
7. cerebrum	**g.** brain
8. aemostasia	**h.** haemostasis
9. polyglobulia	**i.** polyglobulism
10. thrombopathia	**j.** thrombopathy
11. thrombopenia	**k.** thrombopeny

4. Lexical density

This is to measure the density of information through calculating the number of lexical words per clause.

E.g. The <u>implementation</u> of <u>clinical</u> <u>strategies</u> based on <u>optical</u> <u>diagnosis</u> of <u>diminutive</u> (≤5 mm) <u>colorectal</u> <u>polyps</u> may <u>lead</u> to a <u>substantial</u> <u>saving</u> of <u>economic</u> and <u>financial</u> <u>resource</u>.

14

（1）Identify the lexical density of the following sentences

① The rising health problems attributable to obesity are undoubtedly challenging health systems worldwide. _____

② Clinical trials are essential to evaluating EHC innovations and translating them into clinical practice to improve outcomes and quality of life. _____

③ Translation of novel research findings into diverse populations has been surprisingly inefficient. _____

④ We developed the protocol for this systematic review with guidance from previous research. _____

⑤ Consecutive adults undergoing outpatient colonoscopy were considered for inclusion, with enrollment limited to those patients in whom at least one DRSP was detected. _____

⑥ Hybrid effectiveness-implementation design type 3 has a primary focus on implementation outcomes, such as adoption, fidelity, and sustainability.

_____

5. Syntactic ambiguity

Look at the following examples. The underlined expressions are ambiguous.

By adopting a broader range of clinical trial designs, hearing healthcare researchers may be able to extend scientific discoveries to a more diverse population.

In the whole cohort consisting of all epilepsy, the region of the sodium channel subunit gene SCN1A was clearly associated with the disease.

A NMB of zero means that the PECARN rules are no better than the usual care strategy at the threshold of $ 50,000 per QALY.

(1) Identify the syntactic ambiguous expressions in the following sentences.

① The temporal dynamics of normalized synchronization appear to be sensitive to AD progression rate within the limited observation period of a year.

② We assume that these values may be at the extreme of the normal range, or there is the possibility that some factor in the patients' plasma is interfering with the assay.

③ Reduced binding of MDT-15 to NHR-64 might be responsible for the tBOOH sensitivity of mdt-15(rf) mutants.

④ All non-categorical variables were approximately normally distributed, with skew ranging from 1.27 to 1.70.

⑤ Plans also could conceivably incorporate cost sharing or utilization management into the provision of hospice and palliative services, something the traditional Medicare program has not done for the hospice benefit.

⑥ This is consistent with that probability of two recombinations is much less than that of single recombination.

(2) Rewrite the following sentences by using syntactic ambiguous expressions given in the brackets.

① Our results are proved that all five Wnts function to induce expression of elt-5 GATA, to repress expression of elt-3 and to drive aging. (suggest)

② Taken together, it is very cool that the majority of the microglial cell population is long-lived and hence susceptible to aging effects occurring over the animal's lifespan.   (likely)

③ Thus, we also began to see that this kind of training is not adequate to prevent sympathetic overdrive in runners with hypertension.   (suppose could)

④ Some of the strongest familial associations were observed for such less common cancers.   (somewhat)

⑤ This function certainly depends on the microglial cell distribution, process length, and complexity as well as speed of process movement.   (presumably)

⑥ This process will go to oversample large clonal deletions and thus may not yield a true representation of the biological diversity of deletions present.   (tend)

6. Grammatical metaphor

Grammatical metaphor is a substitution of one grammatical class, or one grammatical structure, which is very worthy in scientific genres as a way of expressing objectification and abstraction (Halliday & Martin, 1993; Kazemian et al, 2013).

(1) Identify grammatical metaphor wording in the following sentences.

① People's dissatisfaction with what is, their imagining of how things once were better, or of how things may become, often supports social movements.

② C2 samples harbored an actual microbial community resembling that found in the upper airway or oral cavity.

③ The system equipped with a triple-to-double coincidence ratio (TDCR) counter in the β-channel and a NaI(Tl) scintillation detector in the γ-channel.

④ Dermatologists should be aware of various types of those mucocutaneous manifestations, either common or rare, as well as the management of such conditions.

⑤ The genetic heterogeneity and susceptibility of KD (keloid) vary among different races and ethnicities.

⑥ Fertilization is one of such activities which are people accustomed to do for this purpose from a very long time.

(2) Write grammatical metaphor wording of the following sentences in place of congruent wording underlined.

① For MA plots, the data is dense and points across y axis is shown to reflect the general direction of gene expression changes.

② This may also contribute for us to understand the role of the inflammasome in disease tolerance in bats as reservoir hosts, in contrast to severe pathogenesis in spillover hosts for many high-profile emerging zoonotic viruses.

③ The volatile organic compounds emitted by a fig species are a unique, specific blend that provides a signal to mutualistic wasps that the figs are receptive to be pollinated.

④ The ideal pharmacodynamic parameters of a candidate drug are a rapid onset of action and a fast rate <u>on how to kill and clean the parasite</u>.

⑤ African countries reported that 100% of <u>people who were infected by malaria there</u> were attributable only to P. falciparum.

⑥ In all male mammals, the foundational unit of fertility is the spermatogonial stem cell, which balances self-renewal with differentiation to sustain continuous <u>to produce sperm</u> throughout a male's adult life.

7. Semantic discontinuity

Semantic discontinuity means that writers sometimes make semantic leaps, across which the reader is expected to follow them so as to arrive at a required conclusion.

E.g. In addition, because elasticity coeficients are intrinsically linked to the module kinetics (Brand & Curtis, 2002), and because we only investigated very low and low contractile activities (inducing less than 25% depletion in PCr, activities unlikely to require the maximal oxidative phosphorylation capacity), a decrease in mitochondrial content (or in maximal oxidative phosphorylation capacity) is unlikely to explain the decrease in the elasticity of the energy-supply module found in aged rats. (A) **Therefore, this decrease in the elasticity of the energy supply points toward the existence of an aging-related intrinsic change in mitochondrial function.** (X)

The example consists of two processes, with a logical connection between them. A happened, so X happened.

Task 3B Moves in a medical results section

The results section is generally perceptive to present the findings in an apparently impersonal manner. Kanoksilapatham (2005) proposes four moves in biochemistry research articles, see Table 4.3.

Table 4.3 Biochemistry move/step schemas for a results section

Move 1: Stating procedures	Step 1: Describing aims and purposes
	Step 2: Stating research questions
	Step 3: Making hypotheses
	Step 4: Listing procedures or methodological techniques
Move 2: Justifying procedures or methodology	Step 1: Citing established knowledge of the procedure
	Step 2: Referring to previous research
Move 3: Stating results	Step 1: Substantiating results
	Step 2: Invalidating results

Continued

	Step 1: Explaining the results
	Step 2: Making generalizations or interpretations of the results
Move 4: Stating comments on the results	Step 3: Evaluating the current findings with those from previous studies or with regard to the hypotheses
	Step 4: Stating limitations
	Step 5: Summarizing

Task 4　Build your vocabulary

Work with your partner, match each keyword and phrase to its definition.

Word/phrase	Definition
1. specificity	**a.** a cancer that affects the top layer of the skin or the lining of the organs inside the stomach.
2. overall	**b.** high level or degree; the property of being intense.
3. accuracy	**c.** the colon that located towards the centre of the body.
4. intensity	**d.** the perception that something has occurred or some state exists.
5. conventional	**e.** a drug or another form of medicine that you take to prevent or to treat an illness.
6. deviation	**f.** to bring food from the stomach back out through the mouth.
7. corresponding	**g.** the quality of being specific rather than general.
8. trend	**h.** of or related to the stomach and intestines.
9. detection	**i.** a general direction in which something tends to move.
10. migraine	**j.** including everything.
11. vomit	**k.** to make strong regular movements or sounds.
12. medication	**l.** relating to or connected with the abdomen.
13. pulsate	**m.** similar especially in position or purpose.
14. lesions	**n.** the quality of nearness to the truth or the true value.
15. gastrointestinal	**o.** connected with the colon (= part of the bowels).

16. carcinomas	p. a very severe type of headache which often makes a person feel sick and have difficulty in seeing.
17. abdominal	q. the ability to do the diagnose skilfully without making mistakes.
18. colonic	r. following accepted customs and proprieties.
19. diagnostic accuracy	s. damage to the skin or part of the body caused by injury or by illness.
20. proximal colon	t. a variation that deviates from the standard or norm.

Task 5　Understanding the text moves

Reading 2　Text theme：Artificial intelligence in medical diagnosis

Task 5A　Read the text，and fill in each blank with a proper form of the word in the bracket.

Impact of Artificial Intelligence on Miss Rate of Colorectal Neoplasia
Michael B. Wallace et al

1. In the study period of February 2020 to May 2021，253 subjects were screened，of whom 249 were randomized between the 2 tandem colonoscopy arms，one with AI followed by standard colonoscopy（AI first），the other with standard colonoscopy followed by AI（standard colonoscopy first）（Figure 1）. After excluding 19 subjects who did not at least start one or both the procedures，a total of 230 subjects（116 AI first，114 standard colonoscopy first）at least started both the colonoscopies and were included in the primary analysis population（FAS）. Among these，213 subjects（109 AI first，104 standard first）were included in the PP population. Subject flow is represented in Figure 1. Groups were compared with respect to age，gender，and ____ ____（indicate）for colonoscopy（Table 1）.

2. Quality of the examinations was similar across the study groups（Table 1）. Cecal intubation at the first procedure was achieved in 115（99.1%）and 114（100.0%）cases，with and without AI in the first arm respectively. Bowel preparation was adequate（ie，Boston Bowel Preparation Scale ≥6 and ≥2 in all of the 3 segments）in 220（95.7%）of 230 subjects with no difference between the groups. Mean insertion time and withdrawal times were similar between the study arms（Supplementary Table 1）. The _____（distribute）of the colorectal polyps across each of the 2 arms，for each of the 2 individual procedures according to histology and localization is shown in

supplementary Tables 2 and 3.

Per Polyp analysis

3. **Adenoma miss rate.** The primary endpoint of the study was the AMR. In the FAS population, a total of 493 adenomas (including carcinomas) were detected and removed in the 2 groups. Of these, 246 were removed in the AI first, and 247 in the standard colonoscopy first (Table 2), respectively, and corresponding APC values are provided in supplementary Table 4. In the arm of AI first, 38 adenomas were detected in the second colonoscopy using the standard colonoscopy, corresponding to a miss rate of 15.5% (38 of 246), whereas in the arm standard colonoscopy first, 80 adenomas were detected in the second colonoscopy using AI, corresponding to a miss rate of 32.4% (80 of 247). The logistic mixed model showed a lower estimate for AMR in AI first as compared with standard colonoscopy first (16.6% vs 34.6%, respectively; adjusted OR, 0.38; 95% CI, 0.23—0.62; P<.001); sex, age, and reason for colonoscopy were not statistically _____ (significance) in the model (no influence on the outcome) (supplementary Table 5). The sensitivity analysis using the c2 test confirmed the analysis by the logistic mixed model (OR, 0.38; 95% CI, 0.25—0.59; P<.001). corresponding values of combined ΛPC between the first and second colonoscopy are provided in supplementary Table 4.

4. When subgrouping AMR according to size, among<10 mm adenomas, 35 of 212 were missed in the AI first and 77 of 228 in the standard first, corresponding to a miss rate of 16.5% vs 33.8% (OR, 0.39; 95% CI, 0.25—0.61; P<.001; χ^2 test). When considering adenomas and carcinomas5 mm and 6 to 9 mm, miss rate was significantly lower for AI first in the ≤5 mm group (15.9% vs 35.8%; OR, 0.34; 95% CI, 0.21—0.55; P<.001; χ^2 test), but not for 6 to 9 mm. No difference in miss rate was found for ≥10 mm lesions.

5. When looking at morphology, a total of 246 polypoid-and 245 nonpolypoid-adenomas were removed. Miss rate of nonpolypoid lesions was found to be significantly lower in the AI first (21 of 125, 16.8% vs 55 of 120, 45.8%; OR, 0.24; 95% CI, 0.13—0.45; χ^2 test), whereas there was a numerical decrease in miss rate of polypoid lesions in the AI first, without statistical significance.

6. When subgrouping AMR according to location, this was consistently reduced in the AI first across all colonic locations (Table 2). In detail, proximal colon AMR was 18.3% in the AI first and 32.5% in the standard colonoscopy first (OR, 0.46; 95% CI, 0.28—0.78; P ¼ .004; c2 test), whereas in the distal colon, AMR was found to be 10.8% and 32.1% in the AI first and standard colonoscopy first, respectively (OR, 0.25; 95% CI, 0.11—0.57; P<.001; χ^2 test).

7. When subgrouping AMR according to histology, this was reduced in the AI first for conventional adenomas (15.7% vs 32.2%; OR, 0.39; 95% CI, 0.25—0.62; P<.001; χ^2 test), with no difference for other histological classes (Table 2).

8. Figure 2 shows the forest plot of the AMR overall and by subgroup, _____ (analyse) by the logistic mixed model.

9. **Polyp miss rate.** In the FAS population, a total of 534 polyps were detected in both groups. Among the 261 and 273 polyps detected in the AI first and standard colonoscopy first, respectively, 44 and 85 were missed, corresponding to a PMR of 16.9% and 31.1% for AI first and standard colonoscopy, respectively (OR, 0.45; 95% CI, 0.30—0.68; P<.001; χ^2 test). _____ (correspond) figures according to size, morphology, and location are provided in supplementary Table 6. Supplementary Table 7 reports the results of PMR analyzed by a logistic mixed model: the PMR estimated by the model was significantly lower in the AI first vs standard colonoscopy first (18.1% vs 33.3%, respectively; adjusted OR, 0.442; 95% CI, 0.276—0.708; P< .001). None of the other fixed effects (age, sex, and reason for colonoscopy) was statistically significant.

10. **Mean number of lesions in the second colonoscopy.** When looking at mean number of lesions detected in the second colonoscopy (supplementary Table 8), there was a statistically significant reduction in both the number of adenomas and the number of polyps detected in the second colonoscopy in the group AI first as compared with standard colonoscopy first (mean number of adenomas and carcinomas ± standard _____ (deviate) [SD]: 0.33±0.63 vs 0.70±0.97, P<.001; mean number of polyps ± SD: 0.38±0.68 vs 0.75±0.98; P ¼ .001).

11. The results of the sensitivity analyses on the PP set did not appreciably differ from those of the FAS (data not shown).

Per Patient analyse

12. _____ (detect) **rates in the second colonoscopy.** In the arm AI first, at least 1 adenoma missed at the first passage was detected at the second examination in 29 (25.0%) of 116 patients vs 52 (45.6%) of 114 in the standard colonoscopy first (OR, 0.40; 95% CI, 0.23—0.70; P ¼ .001). When looking at colorectal polyps, at least 1 colorectal polyp, which was missed at the first passage, was detected at the second examination in 33 (28.5%) of 116 patients in the arm AI first vs 55 (48.3%) of 114 in the standard colonoscopy first (OR, 0.43; 95% CI, 0.25—0.74; P ¼ .002).

13. **False negative rate and incorrect surveillance** _____ (intervals). Among subjects who had a first negative examination (no adenomas or carcinomas detected) in the arm AI first, at least 1 adenoma was detected at the second examination in 3 of 44 patients vs 13 of 44 in the standard colonoscopy first, corresponding to false negative rates of 6.8% and 29.6%, respectively, with a significantly lower false negative rate in the AI first (OR, 0.17; 95% CI, 0.05—0.67; P ¼ .006) (Table 3). Among these subjects with a negative first colonoscopy, the mean number (± SD) of adenomas detected at the second examination was 0.09±0.36 in the AI first vs 0.41±0.73 in the standard colonoscopy first, with the difference being statistically significant (P ¼ .006) (supplementary Table 8).

14. Changes in surveillance intervals for patients who had at least 1 colorectal polyp detected in the second colonoscopy are reported in Table 4. As compared with standard colonoscopy first, in the arm AI first fewer subjects had their surveillance interval decreased based on the outcome of the first and second colonoscopies combined in respect to the outcome of the first colonoscopy alone (50.0% vs 35.5%, respectively), with difference between groups showing a numerical _____ (trends) toward a reduction in the arm AI first without reaching the statistical significance (P ¼ .195). No difference in ADR at first or combined procedures was observed between the study arms (supplementary Table 4).

Safety analyse

15. Overall, 17 treatment- emergent adverse events _____ (occur) in 9 patients (6 events in 4 subjects in the arm AI first and 11 events in 5 subjects in the standard colonoscopy first), none related with treatment; among these, 2 events led 2 subjects in the arm standard colonoscopy to discontinue the study. Most of these adverse events were gastrointestinal disorders (mainly abdominal pain, nausea, and abdominal discomfort), followed by general disorders and administration site conditions. No serious adverse events occurred in the study (supplementary Table 9).

From Gastroenterology, 2022, 163: 295 - 304

Task 5B   Read the text more carefully and decide what the moves are.

    1. What're the results of this study?

    2. How do the authors get these results?

    3. How do the authors justify the research results after the research procedures?

    4. What're the steps of stating the results?

    5. What're the differences between the present results and the previous ones?

Section 2   Writing

Task 6   Warm-up writing assignment: Write an effective results section

Task 6A   Grammar and phraseology in medical results sections

    The results section is a concise, brief, and objective summary of the representative data that is logically presented through the core findings, and usually written in the past tense.

1. Sequence

    A clear understanding of the time sequence will improve understanding, prevent confusion, and help your readers to picture and repeat it for themselves. Time sequence means how long each step took and where it occurred in the sequence

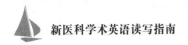

(Glasman-Deal，2009).

(1) Some words and phrases that communicate sequence.

① Before you start observing your results

　　E.g. Based on previous experience，we determined **beforehand that** at least 230 patients were needed to achieve acceptable results；given an anticipated attrition rate a 10%…

② The beginning or first step

　　E.g. We are undoubtedly just **at the beginning** of exploring this field，and there remains an immense amount of work to fully define the relationship between miRNAs and AD.

③ Steps/order

　　E.g. Statistical analysis Normalcy of data was first established using DxA1xAFAgostino and Pearson omnibus normality tests and was **then** analysed by parametric one-way analysis of variance followed by Newman-Keuls post hoc tests.

④ After a short while

　　E.g. Further increase of computational power will **soon** overcome this limitatio.

⑤ At a late/later stage；after a while/longer period

　　E.g. This was performed to maximize the identification of true positive hits，but at the expense of including a large number of false positives，which could **later** be removed in a secondary screen.

⑥ One point/period occurring almost or exactly at the same time as another

　　E.g. In the "cell interactions" tool，when a CCI is selected，"LRI Network" becomes available **when** a specific pair of cell types is selected from the heatmap.

⑦ The end or last step

　　E. g. The urine metabolomes analysed by non-targeted high resolution mass spectrometry were compared **at the end** of the experimental period.

⑧ After the end

　　E.g. **Afterwards**，we respectively introduce research backgrounds and data sources of three categories，and illustrate their representative approaches as well as evaluation metrics.

(2) Put the words and phrases that communicate sequence into one (or more) of the appropriate items.

Items	The words and phrases that communicate sequence
① before the beginning	after, afterwards, as, as soon as, at first, at that point, at the beginning, at the end, at the same time, at the start, beforehand, before long, earlier, eventually, finally, firstly, formerly, immediately, in advance, in the beginning, in the meantime, in the end, initially, just then, lastly, later, later on, meanwhile, next, once, originally, previously, prior to, secondly, shortly after, simultaneously, soon, straight away, subsequently, then, to begin with, to start with, towards the end, upon, when, while
② at the beginning/first step	
③ steps/order	
④ after a short while	
⑤ at a late/later stage; after a while/longer period	
⑥ one point/period occurring almost or exactly at the same time as another	
⑦ at the end/last step	
⑧ after the end	

2. Quantity language

Quantity language can be used to replace numbers or comments on numbers.

(1) Some quantity language examples.

① Increase the size/quantity

E.g. **Substantial** evidence indicates that disrupted neuronal calcium homeostasis is an early event in AD that could mediate synaptic dysfunction and neuronal toxicity.

② Reduce the size/quantity

E.g. The exclusion of the patient with the major protocol deviation had a **negligible** effect on the between-group results.

③ Emphasize how big/small/high/low the size/quantity

E.g. The main strength of our study is a comprehensive set of clinical and correlative data that show safety and **exceptionally high** rates of responses with the combination of ibrutinib and rituximab in patients with CLL who have high-risk disease features.

④ The size/quantity is similar/close to another

E.g. Similarly, both total EGFR protein (Fig. 4F) and EGFR cell surface expression (Fig. 4G) were found to be **approximately** halved in the presence of pre-miR-7 transfections.

⑤ A reluctance to commit oneself to an interpretation of the size/quantity

E.g. **In some cases** the puncta seemed to be at interfaces between two supporting cells, but the possibility that puncta were at a hair cell-supporting cell junction could not be ruled out by epi-fluorescence alone.

(2) Put the words and phrases that communicate quantity language into one (or more) of the appropriate items.

Items	The words and phrases that communicate quantity
① Increase the size/quantity	a great deal（of）, a few, a little, a number（of）, appreciable, appreciably, (higher/lower) approximately, as many as, as few as, at least, barely, below, by far, close (to), considerable, considerably (higher/lower), easily (over/under), even (higher/lower), exceptionally (high/low), extremely (high/low), fairly (high/low), far (above/below), few, fewer (than), greater (than), hardly infinitesimal, in some cases, just, just (over/under), less, little, marginal, marginally (higher/lower), marked, markedly, moderate, more (than), most, much, nearly, negligible, noticeable, noticeably, numerous, only, particularly, plenty, practically, quite reasonably, relatively, significant, significantly, slight, small, so (high/low), some, somewhat, substantial, substantially, to some extent, under, upwards of, virtually, well (under/over)
② Reduce the size/quantity	
③ Emphazise how big/small/high/low the size/quantity	
④ The size/quantity is similar/close to another	
⑤ A reluctance to commit oneself to an interpretation of the size/quantity	

3. Phraseology in a medical results section

（1）Reference to aim，research questions or method

This analysis **aimed to** detect differences in late radiation toxic effects between treatment groups and therefore did not include the 10-week post-radiotherapy assessment，which assessed acute symptom.

The purpose of physical examination in female patients with cancer or cancer history and sexual function concerns is to identify and inform the patient of normal and abnormal findings and to determine the salience of these findings to the patient's presenting symptoms.

Statistical analysis was performed following standardization of specific protein amounts in each sample against NSE，used as a loading control.

Depending on the **question asked**，between 1% and 43% of parents were able to identify the type of product used，and among those，parents were able to supply the name for approximately 70% of products.

The purpose of **the questionnaire was to evaluate** the user experience and preference between the 2D line drawings and 3D body schemas.

All categorical variables **were compared using** two-sided chi-squared tests, and means were compared using independent two-sided t tests.

Regression analysis was used to investigate the relationship between elbow extension (dependent variable) and reach distance (independent variable) for each participant.

We predicted that these differences in secondary antibody binding would make it **possible to distinguish between** the different Hp phenotypes reliably and accurately.

Secondary **analyses examined** the association between psychotic experiences and individual neuropsychological test results.

Heterogeneity of the treatment effect across multiple participating centres **was tested using** a corresponding random-effect linear regression model with site as a random effect.

Paired **t-tests were used** to analyze data involving a single comparison of two level means.

For experiment 1, one-way **repeated-measures ANOVAs were used** to assess changes in performance and EMG data in training sets 1, 12, and 24.

Pearson **correlation coefficient was used** to evaluate the correlation between resting BP and resting MSNA.

According to the results of **ANOVA f-test feature** selection process, two attributes: skewness (3.34) and GLCM homogeneity (3.45) scored the lowest ANOVA f-test scores.

(2) Refer to data in a table or figure

Table 3 shows the joint effect of asthma and rhinitis on the risk of AD.

Figure 2 displays the change in the three alcohol use variables across the four time points of assessments.

Figure 6 displays tumor volume curves for the therapy and the control group.

Figure 5 presents an update of morbidity and quality-of-life endpoints from the RADAR study.

Table 1 provides baseline demographic characteristics of the subjects.

Figure 1 compares the hospitalxA1xAFs overall cesarean delivery rates with the cesarean delivery rates in the United States during the study time period.

Fig. 2 illustrates the two types of BMSCs and the different methods of harvesting these cells.

Equivalence test results **are displayed in Figure 3**.

Participant demographic characteristics **are shown in Table 1**.

As shown in Figure 6, patients who were randomized to topical steroids had a statistically significant but the difference between the groups was not statistically higher IOP at the end of the treatment period than patients significant ($P = 0.42$ for subgroup difference).

(3) Highlight significant data in a table or chart

In contrast, the estimated odds of preterm birth when adjusting for all factors listed **in the Table** were not significantly different between women with a likely diagnosis of PTSD and women with a likely diagnosis of MDE.

This graph shows an excellent correlation between both parameters with a regression coefficient R2 = 0.9764.

The mean ABR amplitude data are shown **in Fig.** 3. There was no difference in the amplitude of wave I, III, V and I—V amplitude ratio between the two ears at baseline.

From this data, we calculated the absolute and percent change between erroneous results and repeats off the original aliquot/tube, as well as absolute and percent change between erroneous result and recollections performed after the erroneous result.

As Table 1 shows, it is only at session 10 that both groups started using the same exact speech processing parameters.

A documentation of patientxA1xAFs pain in the **chart** was found in 57% of all 8447 cases.

Thus, assessing therapeutic CPX improvements through the new multivariate paradigm illustrated in the **Figure is** warranted.

(4) Statements of positive results

The **mean score for** the whole sample for the parent-reported irritability subscale derived from the ODD items of the SNAP was 4.30 (SD^I 2.48) and the median value was 4.

Further analysis showed that many of these correlations are influenced by extreme DNA methylation levels and phenotypic scores exhibited by one male ASD-concordant MZ twin pair.

For the assessment of diagnostic accuracy and **further statistical analysis**, mean values of nerves were pooled even though not all nerves were affected to the same degree.

Two-way ANOVA revealed a significant effect of dose ($F[2, 11] - 32.965$; p less than 0.001), time ($F[2, 11] - 97.666$; p less than 0.001), and a significant interaction of dose and time ($F[2, 22]$ $'9.276$; p less than 0.001.

Strong evidence of underperformance: The probability that the HR was above 1.20 was greater than 75%, or 2.

Differences were considered **significant at** p less than 0.05 based on two-tailed hypothesis testing.

The results indicate that the combined model yields a higher AUC than the fFN test, with a superior specificity and PPV of 100% (Table 3).

There was a modest **positive correlation** between feeling more callous toward people and both percent of clinical effort (Spearman $p = 0.223$, p less than 0.01) and clinical hours worked ($p = 0.208$, p less than 0.01).

A significant **positive correlation** exists between the reduction of leukocyte-derived MP and leptin reduction, TF.

The between-subgroup difference in MMSE **was significant** both at first-year (ti) (p less than 0.005; not given in the table) and second-year examination (p less than 0.001).

(5) Statements of negative results

No increase in CHOP expression was measured.

No difference in leukemic load was observed among the four groups (Figure S2A).

Similar improvements in ambulatory status and mRS scores were also observed after risk adjustment among patients receiving clopidogrel alone or aspirin-clopidogrel dual antiplatelet therapy, although **none of these differences reached statistical significance.**

In contrast to those previous trials, our trial found **no significant reduction** in leg pain following neurodynamic treatment at 2 weeks, and disability was largely unaffected at all time points.

Interestingly, **no evidence was found** for Wnt signaling being involved in cellular or oxidative stress responses during aging.

No significant correlation was found between the OASES-S-D overall score and the total reported duration of treatment ($rho = 0.08$, $p = 0.44$).

Although qRT-PCR of GRM1 (data not shown) and GRM5 (Fig. 4a) showed decreased expression levels in most of the PM cases with increased CGG repeat, **differences were not statistically significant** compared to TD ($p = 0.455$ and 0.115, respectively from two-sample t-tests).

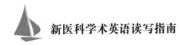

（6）Highlight significant，interesting or surprising results

Interestingly，no evidence was found for Wnt signaling being involved in cellular or oxidative stress responses during aging.

Thus，it is not **surprising** that different dissemination patterns have been seen in patients with MALT lymphomas of various gastric and extragastric sites.

Prediction models built with the full range of variables available are likely to reveal **surprising** relationships that challenge conventional wisdom.

One of the most **surprising** and important results of this paper is how large the welfare gain for society would be compared with the very small cost of compensating kidney donors.

Surprisingly，both drugs inhibited skeletal muscle protein synthesis and prostaglandin production.

This result is **remarkable** with respect to the comparable low sensitivity of confrontation visual field tests frequently used in clinical diagnostic settings.

The **unexpected** finding was that transgenic mice fed the WFD were even more impaired on the spatial memory and NMTS tasks.

Unfortunately，trials combining an anti-VEGF agent or an anti-EGFR agent with gemcitabine and platinum have yielded **disappointing** results，but similar efforts with agents targeting alternative pathways are underway.

（7）Summary and transition

These results suggest that surgery induces neuroinflammation that was inhibited by amantadine.

Taken together，**these results indicate that** ATF6 regulates a subset of UPR response genes，which have been demonstrated or might be revealed to be functioning as pro- or anti-angiogenic factors.

Collectively，**these results show that** lipopolysaccharide alone impaired both contextual and cued fear memory.

Together，**these results provide** the molecular and preclinical evidence for the potential clinical utility of SD70 in MLL leukemia.

Task 6B Literacy skills：Tables，figures，and statistical data
1. Tables

Tables are an effective way of presenting large amount of complicated data in a structured results section.

（1）Basic components and rules of a good table

The essential components of a table should consist of a heading, row and column headers and footnotes. Some rules should be paid attention to: Heading should be short, specific, descriptive, stating the key message to be counted in the table. Each row and column header should be able to interpret what the row/column includes. The footnote should consist of the abbreviations mentioned in the table and any other explanatory notes required (Mukherjee & Lodha, 2016). Captions should be provided clearly, and tell the reader what the table presents. See the example description of Table 4.4.

Table 4.4　Baseline characteristics of patients for the MS disease control analysis

Characteristics	Disease control population($N = 792$)[1]
Mean (SD) age, years	36.2(8.2)
Sex, n(%)	
Male	244(31)
Female	548(69)
Race, n(%)	
White	761(96)
Other	31(4)
Median disease duration, years	6
Number of relapses in prior year, n(%)	
0	9(1)
1	462(58)
2	260(33)
⩾3	61(8)
EDSS score, n(%)	
0	44(6)
1.0—1.5	240(30)
2.0—2.5	261(33)
3.0—3.5	162(20)
4.0—4.5	65(8)

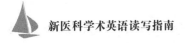

Continued

Characteristics	Disease control population($N = 792$)[1]
5.0	18(2)
⩾5.0	2(<1)
Mean(SD) BPF[2]	0.824(0.022)
Mean(SD) T2 lesion volume, mm³	15 293.8(16 559.2)
Patients with Gd⁺ lesions, n(%)	385(48.6)
Mean(SD) sNfL, pg/mL	16.7(21.1)

BPF, brain parenchymal fraction; EDSS, expanded disability status scale; Gd⁺, gadolinium-enhancing; MS, multiple sclerosis; SD, standard deviation; sNfL, serum neurofilament light chain.

[1] Natalizumab, $n = 537$; placebo, $n = 255$.

[2] Ratio of BPF to total volume within the brain surface contour.

From Table 4.4, we can see:

Heading: Table 4.4. Baseline characteristics of patients for the MS disease control analysis.

Row headers: Mean (SD) age, years, Sex, Male, Female. Race, White, Other, Median disease duration, years, Number of relapses in prior year, n (%)...

Column header: Characteristic Disease control population ($N = 792$)

Footnotes: BPF, brain parenchymal fraction; EDSS, expanded disability status scale; Gd⁺, gadolinium-enhancing; MS, multiple sclerosis; SD, standard deviation; sNfL, serum neurofilament light chain...

(2) Describing tables

Tables and their contents have to be described in the text. Describe the following tables.

For example:

Description of Table 4.5: Baseline characteristics for the 792 (84%) AFFIRM participants who had sNfL measurements are shown in Table 1 (natalizumab [$n = 537$], placebo [$n = 255$]). Baseline characteristics shown in Table 4.5 are typical for a relapsing MS population.

Table 4.5　Univariate analysis: treatment group differences for individual measures of MS disease control

Measure of disease control	Proportion of patients meeting the disease control measure, %		Measures of strength association			
	Natalizumab ($n = 537$)	Placebo ($n = 255$)	OR	ρ-value	Difference	AUC
MRI activity[1]	59.4	13.6	9.3	<0.0001	45.8	0.73
sNfL<97.5th percentile at year 2	90.3	60.4	6.1	<0.000 1	29.9	0.65
Mean(sNfL year 2 and sNfL year 1)<97.5th percentile	88.8	61.0	5.1	<0.000 1	27.8	0.64
sNfL<97.5th percentile at year 2 and year 1	80.7	48.1	4.5	<0.000 1	32.6	0.66
No relapse(1—2 years)	83.2	58.4	3.5	0.000 1	24.8	0.62
No relapse(0—2 years)	63.7	39.6	2.7	<0.000 1	24.1	0.62
No EDSS progression	82.5	73.7	1.7	0.004 4	8.8	0.54
T25FW(<20% worsening)	82.8	76.8	1.5	0.047	6.0	0.53
Annualized BVL < 0. 2% (1—2 years)	45.4	39.6	1.3	0.14	5.8	0.53
9HPT(<20% worsening)	88.4	86.6	1.2	0.47	1.8	0.51
PASAT(<20% worsening)	97.4	97.3	1.1	0.91	0.1	0.50
Annualized BVL < 0. 2% (0—2 years)	32.4	35.5	0.9	0.40	− 3.1	0.52

9HPT, 9-Hole Peg Test; AUC, area under the receiver-operating characteristic curve; BVL, brain volume loss; EDSS, Expanded Disability Status Scale; Gd$^+$, gadolinium-enhancing; MRI, magnetic resonance imaging; MS, multiple sclerosis; OR, odds ratio; PASAT, Paced Auditory Serial Addition Test; sNfL, serum neurofilament light chain; T25FW, Timed 25-Foot Walk.
97.5th percentile derived from Johns Hopkins University normative healthy control data set.
[1] No new or enlarging T2 or Gd$^+$ lesions.

Description:　_____

_____

_____

Table 4.6　Multivariable logistic regression model: Association of measures of natalizumab treatment effect versus placebo

Variable	OR	95% CI	p-value
MRI activity[1]	6.9	4.5—10.6	<0.000 1
sNfL<97.5th percentile at year 2[2]	3.8	2.4—5.9	<0.000 1
No relapse(0—2 years)	1.8	1.2—2.6	0.002 6
No EDSS progression	1.5	0.9—2.4	0.104 3
T25FW(<20% worsening)	1.0	0.6—1.6	0.966 3
PASAT(<20% worsening)	0.9	0.3—2.8	0.806 8
Annualized BVL<0.2%(1—2 years)	0.9	0.6—1.4	0.735 0
9HPT(<20% worsening)	0.8	0.5—1.5	0.521 9

9HPT, 9-Hole Peg Test; BVL, brain volume loss; CI, confidence interval; EDSS, Expanded Disability Status Scale; Gd$^+$, gadolinium-enhancing; MRI, magnetic resonance imaging; OR, odds ratio; PASAT, Paced Auditory Serial Addition Test; sNfL, serum neurofilament light chain; T25FW, Timed 25-Foot Walk. 97.5th percentile derived from Johns Hopkins University normative healthy control data set.

[1] No new or enlarging T2 or Gd$^+$ lesions.

[2] sNfL metric based on largest sample size.

Description:
_____
_____
_____

Table 4.7　Best-fitting three-variable multivariable logistic model predicting natalizumab versus placebo

Variable	OR	95% CI	p-value
MRI activity[1]	7.2	4.7—10.9	<0.000 1
sNfL<97.5th percentile at year 2	4.1	2.6—6.2	<0.000 1
No relapse(0—2 years)	2.1	1.5—3.0	<0.000 1

CI, confidence interval; Gd$^+$, gadolinium-enhancing; MRI, magnetic resonance imaging; OR, odds ratio; sNfL, serum neurofilament light chain. 97.5th percentile derived from Johns Hopkins University normative healthy control data set.

[1] No new or enlarging T2 or Gd$^+$ lesions.

Description:
_____
_____
_____

2. Figures

Figures give a visual key which is usually appealing to the reader. Figures may range from simple line diagrams to scatter plots and radiographs/images. Requirements for writing figures are as follows:

- Make a deliberate choice early in the writing process on which key findings to present in figures.
- The title should reflect what is shown.
- Ensure that tables/figures are self-explanatory.
- Do not repeat information from tables/figures in the text but emphasize the important findings.
- Design figures to make them clear and easy to read.
- Start each table/figure on a new page, after the reference list.

（1） **Graphs/data chart:** Data charts can effectively summarize numerical data for better presentation.

① **Bar charts:** Bar charts may be horizontal or vertical. The height or length of the bars represents the measurement. Describe the following bar charts.

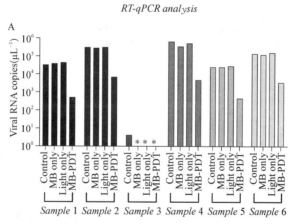

Figure 4.3   Effect of in vitro MB-aPDT treatment in SARS-CoV-2 patient-derived samples

（A） RT-qPCR analysis of 6 samples treated with MB-aPDT （10 min incubation at 10 μM and 30 J c m $-$ 2）, together with control untreated and light-only or MB-only controls.

Description: Six patient-derived samples containing SARS-CoV-2 in universal transport media were treated with MB-aPDT. A signifcant reduction in the viral load of up to ～ 2 Logs as measured by RT-qPCR was observed in all samples treated with MB + light （Fig. 4.3） compared to the control groups （$P < 0.05$ for all）.

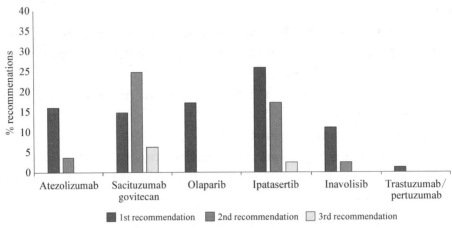

Figure 4. 4   Trial design of COGNITION and COGNITION-GUIDE and preliminary arm assignment of analyzed patient

Hypothetical arm assignment of high-risk patients within COGNITION-GUIDE according to molecular tumor board（MTB）biomarker assignment（n 1/4 81）. AKT，protein kinase B；COGNITION，Comprehensive assessment of clinical features，genomics and further molecular markers to identify patients with early breast cancer for enrolment on marker driven trials；COGNITION-GUIDE，Genomics-guided targeted post neoadjuvant therapy in patients with early breast cancer；eBC，early breast cancer；HER2，human epidermal growth factor receptor 2；PARP，poly（ADP-ribose）polymerase；pCR，pathological complete response；PD-L1，programmed death-ligand 1；PI3K，phosphoinositide 3-kinase；Sacituzumab Gov.，sacituzumab govitecan；Tras./Per.，trastuzumab/pertuzumab；TROP2，Tumor-associated calcium signal transducer 2.

Description：
_____
_____
_____

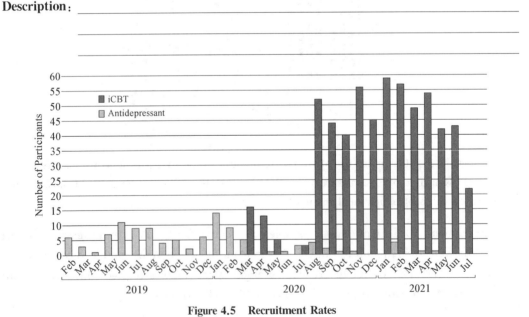

Figure 4.5   Recruitment Rates

Number of participants recruited from each arm from February 2019 to July 2021. The antidepressant arm launched frst，initiating recruitment in February 2019. Paid recruitment efforts were focused on a 13-month period from that date to March 2020，when the iCBT arm commenced. The iCBT arm was initiated in March 2020 via Aware Ireland，and in August 2020 recruitment began through Talking Therapies，Berkshire，South London，U.K.

Description: _____

_____

_____

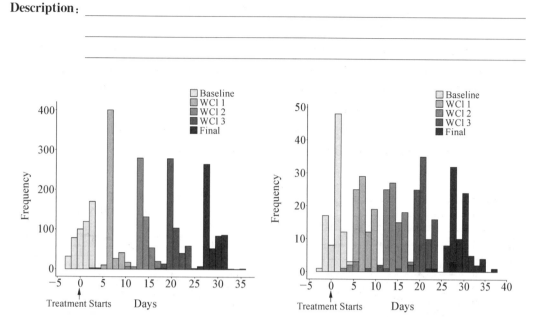

Figure 4.6 Distributions of overlapping completions dates of each study section for (A) the iCBT arm and (B) the antidepressant arm

Day "0" depicts treatment start date.

Description: _____

_____

_____

② **Line plots:** Line plots are good for showing the performance of two or more groups in different conditions that the values of the x variable have their own sequence. Describe the following line plots.

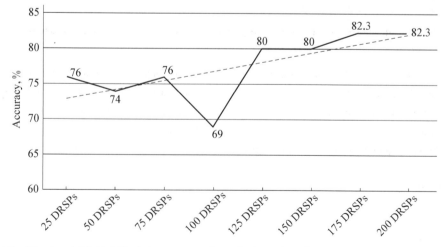

Figure 4.7 The trend (dotted line) in accuracy through the series of consecutive diminutive rectosigmoid polyps evaluated by nonexperts. DRSP, diminutive rectosigmoid polyp.

Description：As far as accuracy was concerned，no differences were observed for experts
（92.0%，95% CI 80.7%—97.7% vs. 90.0%，95% CI 66.2%—89.9%），whereas a trend
toward an increase was observed for nonexperts（74.0%，95% CI 59.6%—85.3% vs.
88.0%，95% CI 75.6%—95.4%）. Interestingly，the AI-assisted NPV of the last 50
DRSPs evaluated by nonexperts met the PIVI-1 threshold（95.2%，95% CI 76.2%—
99.85%）and was similar to the NPV calculated for the last 50 DRSPs evaluated by
experts（93.9%，95% CI 79.7%—99.2%；. The trend of accuracy through the series of
consecutive DRSPs evaluated by nonexperts is shown in Figure 4.7.

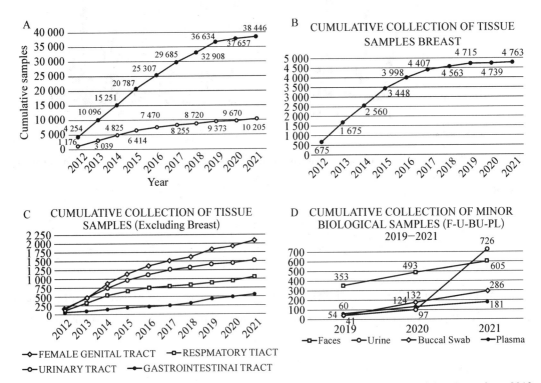

**Figure 4.8   Biobank cumulative collection of biospecimens at the European Institute of Oncology，from 2012
to 2021.**

Cumulative collection of（A）tissue samples（orange curve）and blood with serum samples（blue curve）；
cumulative collection of（B）breast tissue samples（red curve）；cumulative collection of（C）ovary tissue
samples（green curve），prostate（grey curve），lung（light blue curve），and colon tissue samples（yellow
curve）. From 2019 to 2021，cumulative collection of（D）additional biological samples：feces（blue
line），a buccal swab（pink line），plasma（light green line），and urine（violet line）.

Description：_____

_____

_____

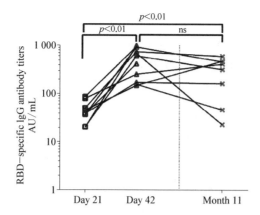

Figure 4.9　Humoral response to BNT162b2

Kinetics of RBD-specific IgG antibody titers before（D21）and 3 weeks（D42）after the second BNT162b2 dose and 3 weeks after an anamnestic dose（Month 11）in vaccinated individuals. Each dot represents a serum sample.

Description： _____

_____

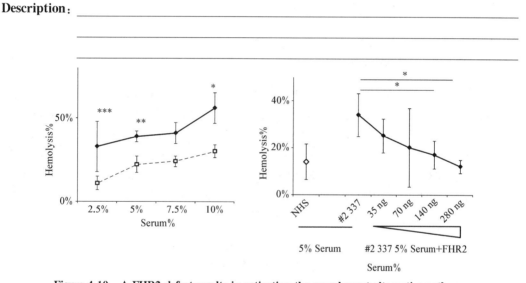

Figure 4.10　A FHR2 defect results in activation the complement alternative pathway

（A）Lysis of guinea pig erythrocytes. Guinea pig erythrocytes were incubated with increasing concentrations （2.5%，5%，7.5%，or 10%）of patient serum HR♯2337（filled rhombus）or NHS（open square）. Lysis was determined by measuring the absorbance of released hemoglobin at 414 nm. The patient's serum induced more erythrocyte lysis（33%，39%，41%，and 56%）than NHS（11%，22%，24%，and 30%）. The difference was statistically significant at serum concentrations of 2.5%，5%，and 10%. The results are mean ± standard deviation（SD）of three independent experiments. * $p < 0.05$，** $p < 0.01$，*** $p < 0.001$.（B）Guinea pig erythrocytes were incubated with 5% NHS（open rhombus）or 5% HR♯2337 serum（filled rhombus）alone or enriched with increasing amounts（35 ng，70 ng，140 ng，or 280 ng）of recombinant FHR2. The addition of recombinant FHR2 reduced erythrocyte lysis from 34% to 12%. The results are mean ± SD of three independent experiments. * $p < 0.05$.

Description： _____

_____

_____

③ **Scatter plots**: Scatter plots can be used to illustrate measurements on two or more relative variables; the values of the variables on the y-axis are consistent with the values of the variable plotted along the x-axis. Describe the following scatter plots.

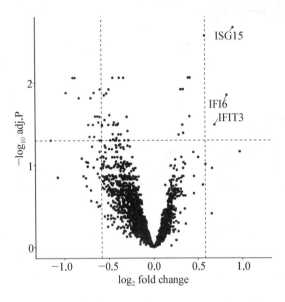

Figure 4.11　Innate antiviral immune response induced by dual mRNA BNT162b2 immunization Volcano plot of the differentially expressed genes on D24 compared to D21 (p.adj<0.05 and Fold Change>1.5 for the upregulated genes, p.adj<0.05 and FC<1.5 for the downregulated genes). Three genes were upregulated (IFI6, IFIT3, ISG15), all involved in antiviral immunity and type I interferon pathways.

Description: We first performed bulk mRNA sequencing of whole blood samples from 15 individuals collected on Days 21 and 24. Four out of thirty samples did not pass quality control and were removed from the analysis. On D24 in comparison to D21, 3 genes (IFI6, IFIT3, ISG15) were found upregulated (p.adj<0.05 and fold change (FC)>1.5) and 18 (AC104389.5, ALPL, BASP1, CHI3L1, CSF2RB, CXCR2, GCA, KCNJ15, MGAM, MME, NAMPT, NIBAN1, NKX3-1, RGS2, SEC14L1, ST20-MTHFS, SVBP, THBD) downregulated (p.adj<0.05 and FC<1.5).

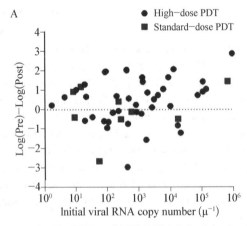

Figure 4.12　Efect of MB-aPDT on SARS-CoV-2 infectivity in clinical samples
(A) Change in viral RNA copies following nasal aPDT vs. pre-treatment load in the same nostril, as measured by RT-qPCR. Black circle 72 J cm − 2, blue square 36 J cm − 2.

Description: _____

_____

_____

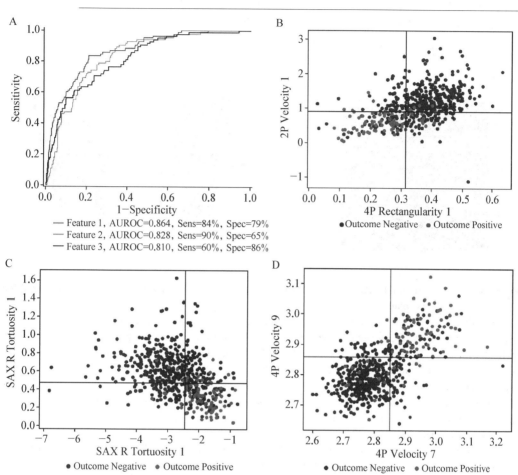

Figure 4. 13   Disease Stratification and Classification Capabilities (A) Example receiver-operating characteristic (ROC) curves of 3 selected features

Feature 1 1/4 A2C at stress rectangularity feature 1, Feature 2 1/4 A4C at stress velocity feature 14, Feature 3 1/4 SAX at rest elliptical variance feature 1. (B to D) Plots of feature values with individuals who had positive clinical outcome colored green and negative outcomes colored orange to demonstrate capability of individual model features to differentiate outcome. Vertical and horizontal lines indicate example cutoff values for disease classification, optimized for balanced sensitivity and specificity. (E) Performance of the artificial intelligence-based classifier on training and independent validation data sets based on ROC curves. Disease stratification is based on an ensemble model built from 31 of the novel features. Feature nomenclature for (B to D): Feature names begin with an indication of the view and stage of the stress echocardiography examination (4P 1/4 A4C view at stress, SAX_R 1/4 parasternal short-axis view at rest), followed by the measurement (eg, rectangularity, tortuosity, velocity). AUROC 1/4 area under the receiver-operating characteristic curve; CAD 1/4 coronary artery disease; Sens 1/4 sensitivity; Spec 1/4 specificity.

Description: _____

_____

_____

④ **Photographic images**: These images are used to document clinical photographs observations of patients, which include radiographs, ultrasonography images, CT scan/MRI scan images, radionuclide studies; intra-operative findings; surgical specimen; pathology images-cytopathology, histopathology, special stains, immunohistochemistry, etc. Describe the following photographic images.

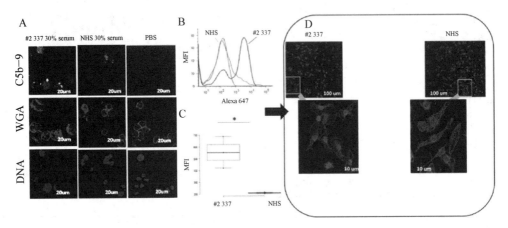

Figure 4. 14   Low serum FHR2 levels result in enhanced C5b - 9 deposition on HUVECs, modifying cell morphology

(A) HUVECs incubated with 30% HS♯2337 (Laser Scanning Microscopy, LSM) showed greater deposition of C5b-9 (green fluorescence) than cells that were incubated with 30% NHS. Nuclei were stained with 4′, 6-diamidino-2-phenylindole (DAPI) (blue fluorescence). The intact membrane was stained with wheat germ agglutinin Texas Red (WGA) (red fluorescence). Scale bar, 20um. A result representative of three independent experiments is shown.

(B) Fluorescence-activated cell sorting (FACS) confirmed the results obtained with LSM. HUVECs incubated with 30% patient serum lacking FHR2 showed greater C5b - 9 deposition than HUVECs incubated with NHS. MFI, mean fluorescence intensity.

(C) The boxplot displays the Mean Fluorescence Intensity (MFI) of HUVEC incubated with either the patient's serum (white) or NHS serum (grey). Data for the triplicate experiments is shown. * $p<0.05$.

(D) HUVECs were incubated with HS♯2337 or NHS. Cell morphology was determined by examination of WGA fluorescence using Laser scanning microscopy. Cells exposed to HS♯2337 are retracted, losing their typical extended shape, and have more intracellular inclusions. Scale bar 100 mm and 10 mm.

Description: As shown in the figure, C5b - 9 fluorescence was intense and diffuse on endothelial cells exposed to HS♯2337, was minimal on cells incubated with NHS, and was absent on cells incubated with phosphate-buffered saline. Moreover, HUVECs incubated with 30% HS♯2337 presented a loss of the typical shape, and their usual morphology was lost (Figure 4.14D). The results were confirmed by flow cytometry. Endothelial cells exposed to 30% patient's serum showed a C5b - 9 signal 2-fold higher than that observed when incubating the cells with NHS [mean fluorescence intensity (MFI) express in percentage: HS♯2337, 554; NHS, 208].

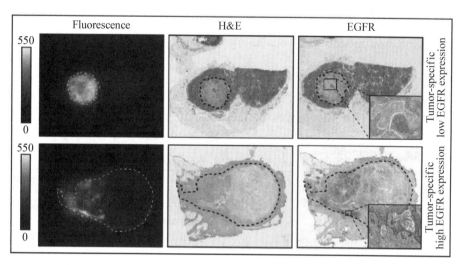

Figure 4.15 Microscopic analysis
Representative images of formal in-fixed LN metastases that were diagnosed on final histopathology. On both fluorescence images and hematoxylin-and eosinstained slides, tumor region is delineated with dashed line. Fluorescence flatbed scanning shows increased fluorescence intensity in tumor deposits, compared with adjacent lymphoid and connective tissue. Although EGFR expression is variable within patients, fluorescence signal is tumorspecific, suggesting that other mechanisms play a role in cetuximab-800CW accumulation. H&E 5 hematoxylin and eosin.

Description: _____

_____

_____

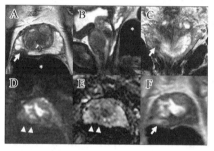

Figure 4.16 mpMRI of a 72-year-old male with a serum PSA of 6.9 ng/mL
Axial (A), sagittal (B), coronal T2WI (C), high b-value DWI (D), ADC map (E), and DCE MRI (F). Patient has a focal lesion (arrow) in right mid peripheral zone which is hypointense on axial (A) and coronal (C) T2WIs, and has a focal contrast uptake on DCE (F). However, due to large amount of rectal gas, visible on axial and sagittal T2WIs (asterisk), high b-value and ADC map images are distorted and lesion cannot be visualized (arrowheads). Targeted biopsy of the lesion revealed a Gleason grade 7 (3 + 4) prostate adenocarcinoma.

Description: _____

_____

_____

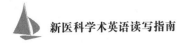

Task 7　Writing task：Build a model

Task 7A　Common models and vocabulary in a medical results section

1. Common models of writing medical results

Several models of scientific writing methods have been presented in Task 3. Nwogu（1997）modified the moves in methods of medical research paper based on Swales' （1981，1990）genre-analysis model，see Table 4.8.

Table 4.8　Outline of moves in medical research articles （Nwogu, 1997）

Results	Move 1：Indicating consistent observation	Step 1：State the overall observation made in the study.
		Step 2：Report on all other significant observations which impinge on the objectives of the research.
		Step 3：Present information on visuals such as tables, graphs and pictorials by using the passive and present tense forms.
	Move 2：Indicating non-consistent observations，presents negative results	Step1：Identify those results which do not conform with expected outcomes in the study.
		Step 2：Make sure the frequency of occurrence of this move in the data used in this study is low.

Move 1　Indicating consistent observation

Step 1：State the overall observation made in the study

Of the 397 participants randomized to receive TBMI，23 participants were for therapist training only either **at the beginning of the study** or during the trial when a change in staff occurred.

Generally speaking，the initial，fast adaptation rates were similar for all groups.

PPP affected 6.3% of the participants' ability to undertake hobbies，and in 10.0% their ability to sleep；however，**in most cases** these impacts were only rated as mild.

In this multicentre study，we compare AQP4 assay metrics on a mixed cohort of patient and control sera performed by 15 European centres that routinely test for AQP4-antibodies.

Therefore，we compare ultrasound-guided core biopsy with other sampling methods of hypopharyngeal cancer.

It is apparent that the items do address a range of issues，including a speaker's impressions about fluency as well as knowledge about stuttering.

The majority of subjects had tumor content of over 90%.

The data of the evaluation of the main variable that is body weight both in the Placebo group and in the Test Group were evaluated and taken into consideration both at the baseline (T0) and after the study period (T1).

However, **the overall response was** less than that seen with transplanted mice not treated with DT, where DCs presenting antigen both directly (donor derived) and via acquisition (recipient DCs) were present.

We obtained expression data using Affymetrix Exon 1.0 ST arrays, which target 270,366 human exons, and Nanostring nCounter gene expression, which allows direct detection of RNA molecules.

Step 2: Report on all other significant observations which impinge on the objectives of the research

There were **no statistically significant difference**s in basic information such as age, gender, and length of stay in the two groups.

Post intervention, the thirst intensity in the intervention groups **was significantly lower than** that of the control group ($p < 0.001$).

Using the sip feed method, NB, PS, and hydroxylation **were significantly increased with** ingestion of protein ($p < 0.05$) during the postprandial period, regardless of amount of protein ingested.

We **obtained primary outcome** data for 114 (97%) participants.

The primary endpoint was met: per patient, the proportions of positive scans rated by the three readers were 67%/67%, 65%/65%, and 73%/70% for ^{18}F-PSMA-11/^{68}Ga-PSMA-11 PET/CT. The miPSMA expression score was higher for ^{18}F-PSMA-11 than for ^{68}Ga-PSMA-11 for the reference reader.

Both groups **were identically matched for** demographics, comorbidities, and indication for LAAO.

Accelerated biodegradation occurred between 31 and 52 weeks, resulting in 82% of implants absent or $\leqslant 25\%$ of initial size by 52 weeks.

However, our findings **revealed significant decreases in** REV-ERBα gene expression ($p = 0.048$) and increases in the REV-ERBα/BMAL1 ratio ($p = 0.040$) compared to baseline in PBMCs isolated from this cohort.

Step 3: Present information on visuals such as tables, graphs and pictorials by using the passive and present tense forms

Histopathological and Immunofluorescence Evaluation Representative photomicrographs of H & E-stained; hippocampal sections **are shown in** Figure 2.

The table **shows** the number of genes expected to overlap between lists of relevant sizes, the number of genes that actually overlap, and P-values (FisherxA1xAFs exact test) indicating significance of said overlap.

Fig. 1 **shows** cumulative free (stroke) survival curves in subjects in the control group(A) and in the Mediterranean diet intervention groups (B).

Simple slopes analysis, **shown in Fig.** 2, **indicated that**, among high reward/low relief drinkers, those treated with naltrexone (relative to placebo) reported significantly less desire to drink over time, $B(SE) = 1.49 (0.45)$, $p = 0.001$, whereas there was no association between receiving naltrexone and desire to drink over time among the other phenotypes (all $p \geqslant 0.26$).

Table 2 **lists** metabolic parameters prior to, and at the conclusion of, the 9 months of treatment.

Gray matter volumes of the trial patients were increased by a mean of 0.3% on an annualized basis (**Supplementary Table** 1).

Between 6 February 2019 and 22 October 2020, a total of 42 patients were enrolled and underwent leukapheresis (**Extended Data Fig.** 1 **and Extended Data Table** 1)

As the results indicated, the osteoclasts had complicated connections with all types of immune cells and osteoblasts (**Fig.** 9A, 9B).

Process and store samples in the biobank, as **presented in Figure** 3.

Table 1 **presents** baseline characteristics of the randomized patients.

Move 2   Indicating non-consistent observations, presents negative results
Step 1: Identify those results which do not conform with expected outcomes in the study

The present findings **did not reveal** significant differences in movement coordination between the AWS and control groups for simple vs. complex nonwords.

It should be noted that current stroke scales are predominantly designed to detect deficits related to stroke in the anterior circulation but are largely insensitive to posterior circulation stroke.

These **unexpected** results highlight the potential complexity of food-food interactions and the potentially unexpected ways in which diet may influence AD progression.

This was an **unexpected** finding, as it was previously shown that Col2. 3 + osteoblasts constitute a niche for lymphoid progenitor cells in the bone marrow.

Although these symptoms are not **unimportant**, the main impact of vitiligo is its visual appearance, so we have not sought to incorporate any physical symptom components into the scale.

Step 2: Make sure the occurrence frequency of this move in the data used in this study is low

However, multivariate analysis indicated HE S as a risk factor only in patients with **abnormal** renal function (total patients OR, 1.2; 95% CI, 0.7'2.2.

Unfortunately, expression of both end-3 and sdz-26 is quite **low** even at day 2 of adulthood, which makes them very poor markers to study the function of Wnt signaling activity all throughout aging process.

These CNVs were, however, not attempted replicated, due to a very **low frequency** (below 1%) in the LLS sample.

Other cells, including dendritic and NK cells, are also crippled, resulting in poor cell cytotoxicity and **low levels** of antiviral cytokine production.

The use of statins and aspirin, which reduce mortality in patients with CAD, was **low** in our patients.

Our results suggest that at **low** levels of screen-detected DCIS, up to 1.

2. Vocabulary in the medical results section

(1) Revise the research purpose of existing research

As discussed previously, this syndrome is common following surgery, but also can occur in up to 42% of medically ill, nonsurgical patients.

As mentioned earlier, genomics has provided us with the unprecedented capability to identify numerous mutations in cancer genes, some of them more frequent than others.

As reported in our Results, we found no significant correlation between the BRAFV600E mutation and gender, multifocality or extrathyroidal extension.

To pursue this issue, **we examined** the mRNA expression levels of these genes using real-time quantitative PCR with RNA samples extracted from post-mortem subject specimens...

It is important to reiterate that these studies (13,14,27) used lower limb exercise interventions whereas CSE was measured from a nonexercised upper limb muscle.

Our purpose was to use DT imaging and graph theory approaches to explore the brain structural connectome in pediatric PTSD.

Therefore, **we investigated** whether polymorphisms in the TNF block are associated with pain intensity in black Southern Africans with HIV-SN.

To test this hypothesis, **we investigated** the contribution of the rs2952768 SNP to the vulnerability to substance dependence in additional subjects with METH dependence, alcohol dependence and eating disorders.

(2) General overview of results

In general, these studies have focused on middle-aged individuals and have emphasized risk over a limited term, often just 5- or 10-year periods (e.g., Assmann et al., 2002).

In all cases, statistical significance of the data was set at p less than 0.05.

Our local, regional, and international networks were very useful in bringing together scholars from the Arab world **in the main**, sometimes in collaboration with international scholars with previous experience in under taking research in the region.

In this article, **we evaluate** the 4-, 12-, and 24-week assessments of the composite primary efficacy endpoint.

It is apparent that there is more heterogeneity for NSOI compared to the better defined entities.

It is evident from visual field and imaging studies and, to a lesser extent, visual electrophysiological studies, that the timing of the testing relative to a migraine (ictal, interictal, duration post-migraine) can influence the results of clinical tests in people with migraine.

On the whole, there is a broad consensus that tomosynthesis in addition to FFDM may be beneficial in the accuracy of cancer detection.

We obtained aggregated screening data for 5 243 658 women screened between April 1, 2003, and March 31, 2007.

（3）Invitation to vie results

These data coincide with the downregulation of EGFR mRNA and protein in aged fibroblasts as seen in **Fig** 1.

As shown in **Fig.** 2A，B，E，F，the treatment of A172 cells with LY294002 or H89 abrogated the PGE2- or forskolin-induced phosphorylation of NF-kB at the sites of Ser 536 and Ser 276，respectively.

As can be seen in Fig. 2B and C，this decrease in the elasticity of the energy supply in aged rats is mainly the result of a greater relative drop in PCr in response to the increase in stimulation intensity from the reference steady state...

Module ［Fig. 2F］ **contains** several mitochondrial factors and enzymes，like，for instance，the mitochondrial transcription termination factor MTERF...

In parallel，Fig. 6 **demonstrates** that harm mediated by hypertension and obesity accumulates from ages 35 to 65，while mortality risk from blood glucose accumulates from ages 58 to 87.

（4）Specific/key results in detail

This result therefore indicates a **decrease** in mitochondrial content with muscle aging.

Our results **expand** on our previous study35 that evaluated the postintervention efficacy of online problem-solving interventions for management of executive function after pediatric TBI.

However，the diagnostic efficiency of SIRT1 to detect frailty was **higher** as compared to SIRT3.

The late stage constriction rate was **unaffected** by age in the 2 C3 strains.

Other synaptic constituents such as Vglut3 and Rab3 proteins are **unchanged** in rbc3a mutants.

These values **match** the expected concentrations within the limits of uncertainty due to the stochastic effect associated with sampling of a dilute solution.

The scratching behavior **peaked** at approximately 10 to 20 minutes in the morphine 0.1 nmol group and at approximately 0 to 10 minutes in the morphine 0.3 and 1.0 nmol groups，and the number of scratches decreased after these times in all the groups （Fig.1B）.

Moreover, before their appearance as clinical phenotypes, cardiovascular diseases are **preceded** by intermediate phenotypes, among which are high concentrations of plasma lipids, such as LDL-cholesterol and triglycerides, hypertension, high fasting glucose or type 2 diabetes, obesity, etc.

The PBV/Vd circ ratio **remained constant** during all stages of hypo- and hypervolaemia (mean values between 0.20—0.22).

(5) Comparisons with other results

The AEs that were categorized prior to study enrollment were characterized **as anticipated** events, and any other event recorded was classified as an unanticipated event.

As expected, the predictive ability of most of the parameters under investigation declines as the overall predictable mortality (measured by the focal exam trace from Fig.2) declines.

In particular, the dose-dependent effects illustrated in Fig. 6 confirm that the IGF-1R $+/-$ mouse is a model of increased longevity **as predicted by** mutations of IGF-1R homologues in invertebrates.

Similarly, **as reported by** researchers investigating performance outcomes for CI-SSD recipients, hearing performance progress is observed to be a function of postimplant listening experience, especially for speech tests performed in spatially separated signal and noise conditions.

These results are **consistent with** our deduction that RNAs produced from a transcription site can enter another transcription site to form RNA subpopulation and that the local distribution of RNAs has preference in a cell nucleus.

These data are **contrary to** prevailing theory that age-related loss of muscle mass is caused by an increase in the ubiquitin proteasome system.

Our findings **corroborate** earlier suggestions that chaotic lifestyle is associated with difficulty adhering to GDM care and thus is associated with poor glycemic control.

The emotional VoiSS subscale was found to **correlate** most strongly with HADS anxiety (0.68, P less than 0.001) and HADS depression (0.62, P less than 0.001).

We did not proceed to the secondary analysis for the patient-focused intervention because we did not **disprove** the null hypothesis for the primary outcome measure.

（6）Problems with results

　　The results show a statistically **insignificant** difference compared with the general population [SIR 0.88（0.29—2.05）], matched for age and sex.

　　The use of MRI for screening in normal and intermediate risk groups is currently questioned because of high costs, limited availability, use of contrast agent and **less than perfect** specificity.

　　However, the effect of out migration on our results is likely **negligible**, since only about 3.6% of those aged 18—49 years move to another state after living in Florida during the 25 previous year.

　　Testing the cutaneous sensory distribution of the femoral, lateral femoral cutaneous, and obturator nerves is **not always reliable** because the cutaneous representation of these nerves varies considerably among individuals, whereas for obturator nerve, it may be missing.

　　Although the exact regulation of EDA + FN splicing is **not completely clear**, it is known that TGF-p enhances EDA + FN production.

　　Although determining the reasons for participants' inability to demonstrate handling skills 2 weeks following retraining were **beyond the scope of this study**, it may be possible that...

　　Such an ambiguity of existing results may be **caused by** several factors, such as variety of applied stimuli...

（7）Possible implications of results

　　Discrepancies between both studies **could be due to** differences in the intensity of exercise and/or the memory tasks.

　　Decreased afferent responses **could account for** the vestibular dysfunction and the raised auditory thresholds in Rbc3a mutants.

　　This result **implies that** in C. elegans, the Wnt signaling pathway plays a different role in longevity than in development.

　　This result, **indicating that** a change in mitochondrial coupling efficiency is unlikely to explain our in vivo results, may be explained by the fact that...

　　Renal function affects sFLC and **in some circumstances** it can cause a difficult diagnosis when using an automated laboratory assay.

　　It is possible that these results **are related to** a previously unrecognized effect from spinal anesthesia...

It could be speculated that this cancer cell proliferation, reduced apoptosis, and increased migration at the time of surgery, together with subsequent metastasis, could explain the clear separation in survival curves between the volatile inhalational and IV groups seen in this study.

Therefore, **it is conceivable that** the aSNpc pSNpc LC precision of neuromelanin MR imaging techniques in tracking the volume of pigmented brainstem nuclei can be improved further.

It links ageing to a **potentially** detrimental characteristic of these neurons, and since neuromelanin is believed to bind iron and chelate it...

These data **support the idea that** impaired pore formation in glaucomatous SC cells is attributable to increased subcortical cell stiffness.

Interestingly, the Bland - Altman plot for CSA (Fig.3) shows that there is a **tendency** of the USCOM to xA1xAEnormalizexA1xAF, that is, higher values are underestimated and lower values are overestimated.

Yet, **there is evidence for** early relative ease with venous access in humans.

Task 7B Building models and move analysis

1. Build models

(1) Content and writing style of the results section

The writing style of the results should be clear, concise, fluent, and objective. The results section is mostly written in the past tense, without unnecessary use of adjectives and adverbs. The findings are presented without interpretation, recognized as mirroring the methods section.

What you should do (Mukherjee & Lodha, 2016)

- Write the results section in the past tense.
- Structure roughly into: recruitment/response, sample characteristics, primary analyses, secondary analyses, and ancillary analyses.
- Match the results section with the methods section.
- Present findings without interpretation.
- Highlight findings from tables and figures in the text.
- Present estimates with 95% confidence intervals.
- Consider providing additional results in tables and figures as webonly supplementary material.

What you should check（Kotz & Cals，2013）

- Decimal points：Usually one or two places after decimal point are sufficient，be consistent with the format.
- Importance of *P* value：Write the actual *P* value，never state a *P* value as 0.000.
- Choose your words carefully：Be cautious while using the word "significant".
- Confounders：Make clear which confounders were adjusted for.
- Negative results：Always report the negative findings as well.
- Text-table dichotomy：Avoid repetition between text and tables.

（2）Results model in medical research articles

The model of a results section is to summarize the key findings and illustrate the data and analyze the results by utilizing both text and visual aids（i.e.，tables and figures），see Table 4.9.

Table 4.9　Results' Model for Medical RA（Huang，2014）

Move 1：Describe study materials	1. Size of study sample
	2. Length of study period
	3. Associations/correlations
	4. Adjustments to analysis

（3）Build models

EASY-APP：An artificial intelligence model and application for early and
easy prediction of severity in acute pancreatitis
Balázs Kui et al

Results：

Characteristics of the original cohort

1. A total of 1184 patients diagnosed with AP were included in the analysis. Eight hundred and seventy-eight patients（74%）had mild，243（21%）moderately severe and 63 patients（5%）had a severe disease course according to the revised Atlanta classification. 2. There were 26 deaths. 3. With the constructed binary class label，1114 patients（94%）were classified as non-severe，while 70 patients（6%）were labelled as having severe disease. 4. Hence，the data had a highly imbalanced class distribution. 5. The general characteristics of the cohort are detailed in Table 1.

Machine learning models

6. We trained and evaluated the following binary classifiers：decision tree，random forest，logistic regression，SVM，CatBoost and XGBoost. 7. The best performing model was an XGBoost classifier with an average AUC score of 0.81 ± 0.033 and an accuracy of 89.1%. 8. The ROC curve and the corresponding AUC are depicted in Figure 2.

9. Although the size of our dataset is larger than that of previously published studies，we investigated how the performance of the model increases as we increase the size of the training set.

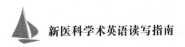

Continued

10. We supposed that the model had not reached its maximal performance and could be further improved with more data (Figure 3).

11. As not all parameters were measured or available on admission, we examined how the performance of the model decreases if it is built from fewer variables. **12**. The AUC values for the models built only on the most important attributes (according to their SHAP values) are shown in Figure 4. **13**. It is clear that performance increased with the number of variables used for prediction, but reasonable performance was obtained with fewer parameters.

14. For binary classification, machine learning models usually only predict a score that can be interpreted as the likelihood of the positive class, here the likelihood of severe AP. **15**. On the other hand, the confidence of the given prediction usually remains unclear. **16**. To assist the physicians in assessing to what extent they can rely on the model's output in decision-making, we also estimated the confidence of the prediction using a bootstrapping method. **17**. The confidence intervals for a selected test dataset of 356 records (30% of the dataset) can be seen in Figure 5.

18. The confidence of the model is greater near the endpoints of the spectrum, that is, when the degree of severity is clearly mild or severe. **19**. On the other hand, the width of the confidence intervals in the mid range is slightly larger.

Explaining the predictions

20. With the help of the SHAP values, the individual predictions of the machine learning model can be explained, and it is possible to measure the global importance of individual features. **21**. The effect of the individual features on the model output and their ranked importance are shown in Figure 6. **22**. The top six most influential features were respiratory rate, abdominal muscular reflex, gender, glucose, creatinine and urea nitrogen level. **23**. The most influential predictors slightly change if the model is trained on other validation cohorts. **24**. The six most influential features regarding all cohorts were creatinine, glucose, respiratory rate, urea nitrogen, white blood cell count and gender. **25**. More detail can be found in Table S9.

26. Using the SHAP values, explanations of three different predictions are depicted in Figure 7. **27**. The features pushing higher the predicted probability of severe AP (compared to the mean prediction, called base value) are shown in orange, and those pushing the prediction lower are shown in green. **28**. Moreover, the length of the bars is proportional to the extent to which the corresponding factor contributes to the prediction. **29**. Note that due to oversampling, the average prediction on the training set does not reflect the prevalence of severe disease. **30**. Hence, it is not the exact SHAP value of a variable that is meaningful in a clinical setting but rather its sign and its relative value in comparison with the other variables' SHAP value.

31. If most parameters of the patient are normal, the risk of developing severe AP is very low (Figure 7A). **32**. The fact that the body mass index (BMI) and glucose level are high, pushes the predicted severity score higher (Figure 7B). **33**. In the case of most parameters being outside the normal range (the patient was older and had a high glucose level, urea nitrogen, BMI, CRP and respiratory rate), the probability of severe disease increased (Figure 7C). More examples can be found in Figure S2.

Validation of the results

34. Our results were validated on external data from four international centres: Alicante, Barcelona, Cluj-Napoca and Liverpool. **35**. Altogether, 3164 cases were included in the analysis. **36**. First, we validated the model's performance by training it on the EASY dataset, and then we measured its performance on the four international centres. **37**. The AUC scores of the model on the Alicante, Barcelona, ClujNapoca and Liverpool data are 0.72 ± 0.036, 0.79 ± 0.039, 0.74 ± 0.041 and 0.77 ± 0.040, respectively. **38**. We found that the performance of the model improves significantly if we supplement the training data with the international datasets; in this case, the cross-validated AUC score is 0.82 ± 0.011 on the EASY dataset, 0.79 ± 0.014 on the Alicante dataset, 0.82 ± 0.020 on the

Continued

Barcelona dataset, 0.79 ± 0.023 on the Cluj-Napoca dataset and 0.78 ± 0.026 on the Liverpool dataset. **39**. Finally, we measured the model's performance on the union of all the datasets; in this case, the cross-validated AUC score was 0.803 ± 0.010. **40**. Further details of the validation cohort and the results of the analysis are available in Supporting Information.

Web application

41. Using the XGBoost machine learning algorithm for prediction, the SHAP values for the explanation, and the bootstrapping method for the estimation of confidence, we have developed a web application (http://easy-app. org/) in the Streamlit Python-based framework. **42**. The application is able to operate if not all the input variables are given; however, at least five input parameters have to be provided. **43**. Although XGBoost can handle missing data, to interpret the SHAP values, we solved this challenge by retraining the model using only the given parameters.

44. The application returns three different plots that show the probability of having severe pancreatitis according to the model (the predicted severity score), the confidence interval of the prediction severity score, the explanation of the decision of the model, and the distribution of the predicted scores made by the XGBoost models. **45**. A prediction in the application is shown in Figure 8.

From Clinical and Translational Medicine, 2022, 12(6), e842

2. Move analysis: Analyze the move structures of the above article

In Sentences 1 – 5, the writers describe the recruitment/response, sample characteristics, and the findings and conclusions obtained in Table 1.

In Sentences 6 – 8, the writers refer back to the methodology.

In Sentences 9 – 10, the writers match the results section with the methods section and make hypotheses to the research.

In Sentences 11 – 13, the writers evaluate the current model with previous model and invite the reader to look at a graph/figure/table, etc.

In Sentences 14 – 19, the writers further match the result of the model with experimental image.

In Sentences 20 – 25, the writers offer the general findings and conclusions and substantiate the hypotheses.

In Sentences 26 – 30, the writers explain the prediction with image, and provide invalidate results and highlight findings from figures.

In Sentences 31 – 33, the writers present findings without interpretation and highlight findings from figures.

In Sentences 34 – 40, the writers use quantity language to support the validation of the findings without interpretation.

In Sentences 41 – 43, the writers show that the writers mention the problems in the methodology and finds solutions to resolve the problems.

In Sentences 44 – 45, the writers estimate confidence intervals, and provide additional prediction in figures and applications of the work.

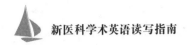

3. The model rebuilt

Moves	Steps
Move 1: Indicating consistent observation	Step 1: State the overall observation made in the study. Step 2: Report on all other significant observations which impinge on the objectives of the research. Step 3: Structure roughly into: recruitment/response, sample characteristics, primary analyses, secondary analyses, and ancillary analyses. Step 4: Match the results section with the methods section. Step 5: Present information on visuals such as tables, graphs and pictorials. Step 6: Present findings without interpretation. Step 7: Use quantity language to support the validation and estimates with 95% confidence intervals. Step 8: Give an account of necessary procedural adjustments made before consistency. Step 9: Consider providing additional results in tables and figures as webonly supplementary material.
Move 2: Indicating non-consistent observations	Step 1: Check decimal points. Usually one or two places after decimal point are sufficient. Be consistent with the format. Step 2: Check importance of P value. Write the actual P value. Never state a P value as 0.000. Step 3: Check the choose of your words carefully. Be cautious while using the word "significant". Step 4: Check confounders. Make clear which confounders were adjusted for. Step 5: Check negative results. Always report the negative findings as well. Step 6: Check text-table dichotomy. Avoid repetition between text and tables.

Task 8 Final assignment: Write an effective results section

Search "Artificial intelligence in translational medicine" or "Artificial intelligence in medical diagnosis" on the internet, or use a sample provided by your instructor. Write an effective results section about artificial intelligence in translational medicine and medical diagnosis using your descriptions of extended tables and figures from the above field.

Your results should contain

- Revising the research purpose of existing research.
- Revising/matching the results section with the methods section.
- Generalizing overview of results.
- Highlighting findings from tables and figures in the text.
- Presenting specific/key findings in detail, without interpretation.

- Comparing with model predictions.
- Issuing problems with the results.
- Presenting possible implications of the results.

Further reading

American Psychological Association. (2022). *Publication manual of the American psychological association* (7ᵗʰ edition). Washington, DC.

Benhammou, Y., Achchab, B., Herrera, F., et al. (2020). BreakHis based breast cancer automatic diagnosis using deep learning: Taxonomy, survey and insights. *Neurocomputing*, 375, 9 – 24.

Bonizzi, G., Capra, M., Cassi, C., et al. (2022). Biobank for translational medicine: standard operating procedures for optimal sample management. *Journal of Visualized Experiments*, (189), e63950.

Calabresi, P. A., Kappos. L., Giovannoni, G., et al. (2021). Measuring treatment response to advance precision medicine for multiple sclerosis. *Ann Clin Transl Neurol*. 8(11):2166 – 2173.

Calabresi, P. A., Kappos, L., Giovannoni, G., et al. (2017). Some aspects of medical english terminology. *Foreign Languages for Special Purposes*, 5 (14), 93 – 105.

Cowan, R. P., Rapoport, A. M., Blythe, J., et al. (2022). Diagnostic accuracy of an artificial intelligence online engine in migraine: A multi-center study. *Headache: The Journal of Head and Face Pain*. 62(7):870 – 882.

Derfus, G., Johal, A. S., Barawi, M., et al. (2022). Impact of artificial intelligence on miss rate of colorectal neoplasia. *Gastroenterology*. 163(1):295 – 304.e5.

Drotar, D. (2009). How to write an effective results and discussion for the Journal of pediatric psychology. *Journal of Pediatric Psychology*, 34(4), 339 – 343.

Faryadi, Q. (2019). PhD thesis writing process: A systematic approach-How to write your methodology, results and conclusion. *Online Submission*, 10, 766 – 783.

Fryer, D. L. (2012). Analysis of the generic discourse features of the English-language medical research article: A systemic-functional approach. *Functions of language*, 19(1), 5 – 37.

Gama, F., Tyskbo, D., Nygren, J., et al. (2022). Implementation frameworks for artificial intelligence translation into health care practice: Scoping review. *J Med Internet Res*, 24(1):e32215.

Glasman-Deal, H. (2009). *Science research writing for non-native speakers of English*. World Scientific.

Gorbalenya, A. E., Krupovic, M., Mushegian, A. R., et al. (2020). The new scope of virus taxonomy: partitioning the virosphere into 15 hierarchical ranks. *Nature*

Microbiology，5(5)，668－674.

Halliday，M. A. K. (2006). *Language of science*（Vol. 5）. Bloomsbury Publishing.

Halliday，M. A. K.，& Martin，J. R. (1993). *Writing science. Literacy and discourse power*. London：Flamer Press.

Halliday，M. A. K.，& Webster，J. J. (2009). *Continuum companion to systemic functional linguistics*. London：Continuum.

Kanoksilapatham，B. (2005). Rhetorical structure of biochemistry research articles. *English for specific purposes*，24(3)，269－292.

Kazemian，B.，Behnam，B.，& Ghafoori，N. (2013). Ideational grammatical metaphor in scientific texts：A Hallidayan perspective. *International Journal of Linguistics*，5(4)，146－168.

Kotz，D.，& Cals，J. W. L. (2013). Effective writing and publishing scientific papers，part iv：methods. *Journal of Clinical Epidemiology*，66(8).

Kui，B.，Pintér，J.，Molontay，R.，et al. (2022). EASY-APP：An artificial intelligence model and application for early and easy prediction of severity in acute pancreatitis. *Clin Transl Med*. 12(6)：e842.

Lee，C. T.，Palacios J.，Richards D.，et al. (2023). The Precision in Psychiatry (PIP) study：Testing an internet-based methodology for accelerating research in treatment prediction and personalisation. *BMC Psychiatry*. 23(1)：25.

Lin，Y.，Yilmaz，E. C.，Belue，M. J.，et al. (2023). Prostate MRI and image Quality：It is time to take stock. *Eur J Radiol*. 161：110757.

Maher，J. (1986). English for medical purposes. *Language teaching*，19(2)，112－145.

Mann，D. L. (2023). Artificial Intelligence Discusses the Role of Artificial Intelligence in Translational Medicine：A *JACC：Basic to Translational Science* Interview With ChatGPT. *JACC Basic Transl Sci*. 8(2)：221－223.

Mukherjee，A.，& Lodha，R. (2016). Writing the results. *Indian Pediatr*，53(5)，409－15.

Papadatou，I.，Geropeppa，M.，Verrou，K. M.，et al. (2023). SARS-CoV-2 mRNA Dual Immunization Induces Innate Transcriptional Signatures，Establishes T-Cell Memory and Coordinates the Recall Response. *Vaccines*（Basel），11(1)：103.

Pires，L.，Wilson，B. C.，Bremner，R.，et al. (2022). Translational feasibility and efficacy of nasal photodynamic disinfection of SARS-CoV-2. *Sci Rep*. 12(1)：14438.

Pixberg，C.，Zapatka，M.，Hlevnjak，M.，et al. (2022). COGNITION：a prospective precision oncology trial for patients with early breast cancer at high risk following neoadjuvant chemotherapy. *ESMO Open*. 7(6)：100637.

Pratt，A. W.，& Pacak，M. G. (1969). Automated processing of medical English. In *International Conference on Computational Linguistics COLING* 1969：*Preprint No*. 11.

Rondonotti, E., Hassan, C., Tamanini, G., et al. (2023). Artificial intelligence-assisted optical diagnosis for the resect-and-discard strategy in clinical practice: the Artificial intelligence BLI Characterization (ABC) study. *Endoscopy*, 55(1): 14 – 22.

Salto-Tellez, M., Cree, I. A. (2019). Cancer taxonomy: pathology beyond pathology. *Eur J Cancer*. 115:57 – 60.

Snyder, N., Foltz, C., Lendner, M., et al. (2019). How to write an effective results section. *Clinical Spine Surgery*, 32(7), 295 – 296.

Stea, E. D., Skerka, C., Accetturo, M., et al. (2022). Case report: Novel FHR2 variants in atypical Hemolytic Uremic Syndrome: A case study of a translational medicine approach in renal transplantation. *Front Immunol*. 13:1008294.

Tatonetti, N. P. (2019). Translational medicine in the Age of Big Data. *Brief Bioinform*. 20(2):457 – 462.

Terranova, N., Venkatakrishnan, K., Benincosa, L. J. (2021). Application of machine learning in translational medicine: Current status and future opportunities. *AAPS J*. 23(4):74.

Upton, R., Mumith, A., Beqiri, A., et al. (2022). Automated echocardiographic detection of severe coronary artery disease using artificial intelligence. *JACC Cardiovascular Imaging*. 15(5):715 – 727.

Visaggi, P., Barberio, B., Gregori, D., et al. (2022). Systematic review with meta-analysis: artificial intelligence in the diagnosis of oesophageal diseases. *Aliment Pharmacol Ther*. 55(5):528 – 540.

Zhang, L., Kopak, R., Freund, L., & Rasmussen, E. (2011). Making functional units functional: The role of rhetorical structure in use of scholarly journal articles. *International Journal of Information Management*, 31(1), 21 – 29.

Unit 5
Reading and Writing a Discussion/ Conclusion Section

The discussion section is the hardest section, and the conclusion is an essential part of writing a medical article. The discussion/conclusion section can be either written separately or combined into one section. Reading and writing "Discussion" and/or "Conclusion" sections in medical articles require a procedure as exact and structured as that concerned about raising questions, choosing materials and methods and producing results for a medical research. Generally, the discussion and conclusion section should: 1) interpret or give meaning to the research results, 2) highlight the real-world relevance of the study findings, 3) address the study's limitations, 4) make the reader understand the researcher's rationale for the study, have a clear answer to the study hypotheses, and appreciate the findings' clinical implications, 5) deduce the major findings and their broader clinical or real-world significance, 6) summarize the study's methods, results, and significance, 7) convey the study's key findings and how they expand the field (Jenicek, 2006; Makar et al, 2018)

Highlight

In this unit, you will

- Learn vocabulary related to artificial intelligence in treatment and artificial intelligence in nursing
- Use suitable expressions and grammatical forms when comparing and contrasting information
- Recognize how argument and critiques are integrated in texts
- Organize move-steps from readings into writings that reflect the purposes of writing discussion/conclusion
- Learn about building an academic vocabulary bank
- Build a model for a discussion/conclusion section
- Write a short comparison and contrast discussion, integrating argument with critiques
- Write an extended discussion/conclusion concerning artificial intelligence in treatment/nursing.

Gearing up

Work in a small group and discuss what you should know before drafting a discussion/ conclusion section or what you should avoid when writing the discussion/conclusion section. Can you add more to the list below?

1. What should you know before drafting?

(1) What are the most important findings of your study?

(2) Did you reject the hypothesis?

(3) Did your findings suggest an alternative hypothesis?

(4) What are the strengths and weaknesses of your study?

(5) Are there any other factors that influenced your findings? What are they?

(6) How are your findings related to those of other relevant studies?

(7) Why are the findings of your study different from those of other studies?

(8) Did you explain unexpected findings?

(9) What assumptions did you make upfront?

2. What should you avoid when writing?

(1) Including too little or too much text.

(2) Including text without structure (open with a narrow focus and then generalize).

(3) Including data not presented in the results section.

(4) Describing detailed aspects of the results.

(5) Relating results to interpretations.

(6) Emphasizing irrelevant and incidental findings (remain focused on the hypothesis).

Section 1   Reading

Task 1   Activating background knowledge

Task 1A   Discuss the following questions

1. What is the main purpose of the discussion/conclusion section?

2. What elements should be included in the discussion/conclusion section?

3. What things should be avoided in the discussion/conclusion section?

4. What is the meaning of the IMRAD in medical papers?

5. What are components of a modern argument in medicine?

Look at Table 5.1 and tick your items, and then share your answers with your

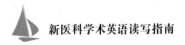

classmates.

Table 5.1   Questionnaire for writing a discussion/conclusion section in medical research (Hess, 2004)

Items	True	False
① One of the purposes of the discussion is to explain the findings and why they are important.		
② The findings of other studies may support your findings, which strengthens the importance of your results.		
③ It is also important to point out how your study differs from other similar studies.		
④ Experimental studies conducted in the laboratory usually do not involve human subjects, but the results may have clinical implications, which should be stated.		
⑤ The best studies in the most prestigious journals have limitations.		
⑥ In some journals the conclusions section is a paragraph or subsection at the end of the discussion, whereas other journals (*RESPIRATORY CARE*, for instance) require a separate conclusions section.		
⑦ The conclusions section may also provide suggestions for practice change, if appropriate.		
⑧ Your interpretation of the results can go beyond what is supported by the data a little.		
⑨ It is important to remain focused on the hypothesis and study results.		
⑩ You can use the discussion section to criticize other studies.		

Task 1B   To help you to read, understand and write discussion/conclusion in medical articles effectively, here are some descriptions in Table 5.2 that you are required to tick.

Table 5.2   Questionnaire for the structure and content of the discussion/conclusion section (Jenicek, 2006)

Structure and Content	YES	NO
1. The Introduction-(Material and) Methods-Results-and-Discussion (and conclusions) format is usually used in medical writing.		
2. Revise and summarize major findings (claims) of the study.		
3. Succinctly remind the reader of the original thesis (statement of the problem) of the study.		
4. Critically appraise the evidence in grounds and its relevance to the study and its claims.		
5. Critically appraise both the supporting and contradictory evidence (if any) in backing and its relevance in connection to grounds and claims).		

Continued

6. Critically analyze and appraise the value, relevance and biological, social and technical（if any）plausibility of the warrant in general, and specifically pertaining to the study.		
7. Assess the link between argument building blocks and the relevance of their content to the final conclusions（claims）.		
8. Present the final conclusions（claims）stemming from the study（or refer to 2）, corroborating with or contradicting the original thesis as stated in 3）.		

Task 2 Understanding the facts and details

Reading 1 Text theme: Artificial intelligence treatment

Task 2A Read the text, and fill in each blank with a proper form of the word in the bracket.

Identification of Determinants of Biofeedback Treatment's Efficacy in Treating Migraine and Oxidative Stress by ARIANNA（ARtificial Intelligent Assistant for Neural Network Analysis）

Irene Ciancarelli et al

Discussion

1. Chronic migraineurs have higher oxidative stress and a lower antioxidant capacity, and the expression of nitrate, nitrite, and nitric oxide reductase genes is significantly higher in migraineurs than in non-migraineurs. In line with these assumptions, our previous results showed, in chronic migraine before biofeedback sessions, decreased SOD and NOx serum levels and increased peroxide serum levels with respect to the levels in healthy control subjects. In our previous study, the lower NO bioavail-ability in migraineurs was explained as a consequence of decreased SOD activity, which probably caused a quicker and more consistent reaction of NO with free- radical species such as peroxides, decreasing the NO level. These data were confirmed by the lack of significant differences in the NOx serum levels, as well as SOD and peroxide levels, between the migraineurs after biofeedback and healthy control subjects. In this study, the ANN analysis validated the efficacy of biofeedback in limiting oxidative processes by improving SOD activity and thus scavenging superoxide anions（Table1）, underlying the role of biofeedback training not only as an efficacious behavioral/ relaxation therapy, but also as a _____（strategies）treatment to reduce the vulnerability of migraineurs to oxidative stress. Moreover, the muscular relaxation induced by biofeedback is promoted by an enhancement of NO bioavailability through the activation of NO pathways. Furthermore, the relaxation-based treatment performed with biofeedback is confirmed to be extremely useful as a therapeutic approach, decreasing the headache-related disability and improving the independence

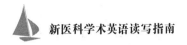

in the activities of daily living of migraineurs, as determined by the ANN analysis of the MIDAS score, which _____ (signify) decreased after the biofeedback sessions, suggesting the potential effectiveness of biofeedback in migraine treatment, as well as in migraineurs abusing analgesic drugs and who have greater compliance with non-pharmacological treatments. The results of our study are in line with the conclusions of the most recent manuscripts, confirming the efficacy of behavioral approaches in headache treatment. Particularly, our results also show that biofeedback, inducing muscular relaxation and modulating biomarkers, represents an efficacious non-pharmacological approach for migraine prophylaxis, as also described in other manuscripts.

2. The main limitation of this study was the small sample size of 20 participants; for each, five variables were assessed at baseline. Further studies should _____ (investigates) more samples. However, despite this small dataset, the ANN achieved good accuracy in predicting

the outcome.

3. With the purpose of interpreting the complex relationship emerging from biological data, as in our study, in order to identify prognostic factors for migraine recovery and disability alleviation, the ANN turns out to be an innovative methodology able to highlight important relationships that simple correlations may fail to identify as statistically significant. The _____ (complexities) of these relationships was, in fact, confirmed by the absence of significant correlations of the pre-treatment variables with the post-treatment MIDAS score. The complexity of these relationships also results from the high number of hidden elements (20 and 15) self-determined by the neural network and needed to predict the outcome. The most important factor useful for predicting the MIDAS score post-treatment was the NOx serum levels, followed by the peroxide serum levels (both assessed pre-treatment). As stated above, there was not a simple linear correlation between these latter two variables and the MIDAS post-treatment; for this reason, there was a need for a more complex algorithm to highlight their influence on this outcome. The accuracy of the ANN was about 75%, with an overestimation of the MIDAS score in most of the remaining cases (25%), as also shown by the frequency distributions reported in Figure 2. The ANN results suggest that a higher level of NO pre-treatment is related to a lower MIDAS score post-treatment, but only if peroxides are in a specific range (116-205 U/mL) _____ (exclusive) extreme values pre-treatment (lower than 116 U/mL or higher than 205 U/mL). For this reason, data analysis with the ARIANNA methodology, despite the high complexity of the neural network (with a total of 35 hidden elements), constitutes a significant opportunity in clinical practice for identifying prognostic factors for the efficacy of therapeutic approaches.

Conclusion

The analysis conducted by using the artificial neural network ARIANNA on the relationship between biomarkers and biofeedback treatment in migraineurs revealed a complex relationship in which the increase in NOx, when serum level of peroxides lies within a specific range, is the most important factor for predicting biofeedback's efficacy in reducing migraines. In conclusion, the perspective of this study is to reiterate the efficacy of biofeedback in the prophylactic treatment of migraines and, above all, to underline that the analysis of biological data with the ANN may represent an appropriate _____ (methodologies) for identifying the predictive factors for therapeutic effectiveness.

From the Journal Healthcare, 2022, 10(5), 941

Task 2B　Read the text more closely. Decide whether these statements are TRUE (T) or FALSE (F).

1. Chronic migraineurs have higher oxidative stress and a lower antioxidant capacity, and the expression of nitrate, nitrite, and nitric oxide reductase genes is significantly higher in migraineurs than in non-migraineurs.　（　）

2. The ANN analysis validated the efficacy of biofeedback in limiting oxidative processes by improving SOD activity and thus scavenging superoxide anions (Table 1), underlying the role of biofeedback training not only as an efficacious behavioral/relaxation therapy, but also as a strategic treatment to increase the vulnerability of migraineurs to oxidative stress.　（　）

3. Furthermore, the relaxation-based treatment performed with biofeedback is confirmed to be extremely useful as a therapeutic approach, decreasing the headache-related disability and improving the independence in the activities of daily living of migraineurs.　（　）

4. Further studies should investigate more samples. However, the ANN does not achieved good accuracy in predicting the outcome.　（　）

5. The complexity of these relationships was, in fact, confirmed by the absence of significant correlations of the pre-treatment variables with the post-treatment MIDAS score.　（　）

6. Data analysis with the ARIANNA methodology, despite the high complexity of the neural network (with a total of 35 hidden elements), constitutes a significant opportunity in clinical practice for identifying prognostic factors for the efficacy of therapeutic approaches.　（　）

7. The perspective of this study is to reiterate the efficacy of biofeedback in the prophylactic treatment of migraines.　（　）

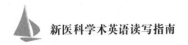

Task 3　Academic literacy skills：Read for specific information

Task 3A　Understand characteristics of medical English

Comparison and contrast is a very common logic pattern in most NEMP articles. The writers need to explain the similarities and the differences when classifying. The logic pattern of comparison and contrast is used to study the tables，figures，and other statistical information.

1. Comparison and contrast

（1）Model：Comparison/contrast discussion section

> **Para. 1.** Our results suggest a role for sNfL levels as a biomarker of neuroaxonal damage and disease activity in the early assessment of natalizumab treatment. Neurofilaments are structural scaffolding proteins of the neurons and are released in response to neuroaxonal damage. [22] Elevated levels of NfL have been detected in the cerebrospinal fluid and serum of patients with MS，and it has been suggested as a prognostic marker for MS. [22] In patients with MS，higher sNfL levels correlated with clinical and imaging measures of disease severity，including brain and spinal cord volume loss. [22 – 25] sNfL levels decrease in patients with MS treated with DMTs. [22-24] Changes in sNfL levels can be easily measured in blood samples with high reliability and sensitivity using recently developed bioassays. [24,26,27] Up-to-date evidence shows that higher sNfL levels may also be an indicator of suboptimal drug response [28] and disease activity when routine clinical and MRI assessment produce false negatives. [29] The integration of sNfL as a blood-based biomarker in MS clinical practice will be dependent on the technical and clinical validation of sNfL as a diagnostic test，improved understanding of confounding variables such as comorbid illnesses and body mass index，and，finally，the establishment of normal age-related reference values. [30] Thereafter，a simple blood test to measure sNfL levels could complement MRI in monitoring the effectiveness of natalizumab and possibly other anti-inflammatory DMTs.
>
> **Para. 2.** Brain atrophy can be seen in the earliest stages of MS and predicts future cognitive and physical disability. [31,32] BVL values depend on the methodology used to generate them. The image analysis techniques，and to a lesser extent the image acquisitions，have a significant impact on volumetric measurements. The optimal threshold for BVL is not yet clear and it is possible that results may change with the use of an alternative threshold.
>
> **Para. 3.** There are a number of limitations of this study，including that it was conducted over 2 years and reflects short term variables such as inflammatory markers. The study findings should be assessed over longer time frames，after which other measures，such as BPF and cognition，may add increased relevance

and stronger contributions to the model. In addition，the data presented are from post hoc analyses of a clinical trial and，although informative，should be confirmed in a real-world setting across a broader range of MS clinical subtypes. In AFFIRM，6% of the patients treated with natalizumab developed persistent antibodies to natalizumab[16]; our sampling did not exclude these patients. Furthermore，this study addresses the value of different prognostic factors in differentiating natalizumab from placebo and cannot automatically be generalized to other treatments with different effect sizes or modes of action. Ongoing studies will add to our understanding of whether patients meeting the criteria defined by sNfL and MRI measurements（new and enlarging T2 and Gd$^+$ lesions）alone will have better long-term outcomes than predicted using the original NEDA measurement.

From Annals of Clinical and Translational Neurology，2021，8(11)：2166–2173.

Writing technique questions

① In which paragraph(s) are the similarities discussed?

② In which paragraph(s) are the differences discussed?

③ How to organize a comparison/contrast paragraph in the above text?

(2) Comparison signal words

It is important to write effective comparison/contrast paragraphs by using appropriate comparison and contrast signal words. Table 5.3 lists some words and phrases used to discuss similarities.

Table 5.3　Comparison signal words

Transition Words and Phrases	
similarly likewise	This suggests that a similar mechanism is underlying both YRV and gene expression differences in flies with different sex chromosome configurations. **Similarly**, we find that genes whose expression is sensitive to rDNA copy number（Paredes et al. 2011）tend to be differentially expressed between karyotypes with different number of Y chromosomes.
also	Remarkably, the expression pattern was **also** retained in a patient-specific manner, even within each subtype.
too	Here **too**, none of the post-endocrine therapy EGFR-amplified tumors harbored known ESR1 mutations that could explain treatment resistance.
Subordinators	
as just as	MSA of CDSs were concatenated and then, **just as** with the whole-genome analysis, variant sites were obtained using SNP-sites and flux estimates were obtained by counting the frequency of each type of change with respect to the reference.
and	OSM **and** OSMR expression levels were also elevated in patients who responded initially to infliximab, but relapsed by week 30 after treatment
both...and	Unfortunately, expression of **both** end-3 **and** sdz-26 is quite low even at day 2 of adulthood, which makes them very poor markers to study the function of Wnt signaling activity all throughout aging process.

Continued

Subordinators	
not only...but also	For instance，LY294002 is an antagonist **not only** for PI3-K but also for Casein kinase Ⅱ（Davies et al.，2000）.
neither...nor	The patient and control groups differed **neither** in age **nor** in level of education.
Others	
like(+ noun) just like(+ noun) similar to (+ noun)	For instance，in Indonesia it was found that older people who engaged in sports had a halved risk of dementia（Hogervorst et al.，2012），which was **similar to** data from the US and other countries（Barnes and Yaff，2011）.
(be) like (be) similar (to) (be) the same as	The NMR structure of chicken cystatin was essentially **the same as** the crystal structure（Dieckmann et al.，1993；Engh et al.，1993）.
(be) the same	...here is a financial advantage to the payor and the patient，and a time savings for the surgeon，provided that long-term outcomes **are the same**.
(be) alike (be) similar	Domains identified by this method **are similar** in size to compartmental domains identified by high-resolution Hi-C（Figure S3H）.
To compare (to/ with)	These results should **be compared** with the histologic analysis of the whole liver explants serving as the gold standard.

（3）Use comparison signal words from Table 5.3 to complete the following sentences.

① From such measurements it is possible to estimate the size of the readily-releasable pool of vesicles corresponding to 10—14 vesicles per ribbon；_____ 280 in mouse IHCs，corresponding to 11 per each of 25 ribbons.

② We propose that MDT-15xA1xAFs function in ROS defense may _____ underlie its lifespan promoting role，perhaps in parallel to mdt-15-dependent lipid signaling.

③ However，the reported accuracies are not for the same datasets，and therefore can not _____ each other.

④ The structures of adjacent regions of chromatin _____ one another Our RNA population model requires that the structures of adjacent chromatin regions are similar to one another.

⑤ Because the latter two categories _____ ，for some analyses we combined them into one category，called generally happy.

⑥ _____ the amount _____the type of HE S administration alone increased AKI incidence by multivariable analysis.

⑦ We hypothesized that resistance to type I collagen proteolysis _____ marks biological aging _____drives it.

⑧ Results NCX3 is cleaved by _____ calpain-1 _____ caspase-3 in cell models of neurological disease (Bano et al., 2005).

(4) Use different comparison signals to write five sentences.

① _____

② _____

③ _____

④ _____

⑤ _____

(5) Contrast signal words

The signal words in the first column of Table 5.4 show concessional relationship, and the words in the second column show an opposition relationship.

Table 5.4   Contrast signal words

Contrast signal words: concession	
Transition words and phrases	
however nevertheless nonetheless still	Several studies have previously reported an increased incidence of testicular cancer among Hispanics, which may be related to a range of risk exposures; **nevertheless**, with such highly effective treatment available, the high rates in these communities raise questions about access to quality care.
Subordinators	
though even though although	**Even though** many studies suggest that Ap imaging using positron emission tomography scanning and Ap levels measurement in CSF and serum may serve as promising methods in diagnosis, the high cost and invasive nature preclude their utility for routine clinical tests.
Coordinators	
yet but	Animals tightly control ROS levels using sophisticated defense mechanisms, **yet** the transcriptional pathways that induce ROS defense remain incompletely understood.
Others	
in spite of (+ noun) despite(+ noun)	**In spite of** this matching, the two subgroups remained incomparable in a number of relevant clinical characteristics, including mechanism of injury, injury severity, and body region injured.

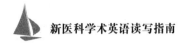

Continued

Contrast signal words: direct opposition	
Transition words and phrases	
on the other hand in (by) comparison in contrast however	In a study using another method of telomere measurement, flow FISH, variance of telomere length did decrease with age, **in contrast** with the presented meta-analysis, but with a markedly lower sample size of 181 compared to a total of 16,384 subjects in the meta-analysis presented here.
on the contrary	There was no association between CMBs and atrophy; **on the contrary**, CMBs were associated with a small increase in basal ganglia and cerebellar volume, for unclear reasons.
Subordinators	
whereas while	These differences suggest a generally slower, less dynamic response to injury in aged microglia, **whereas** young adult microglia rapidly increased their process motility in response to laser injury.
Coordinators	
but	SIRT1and 3 levels decreased in patients with diabetes and hypertension, **but** the levels were even lower in individuals who were frail and had diabetes or hypertension.
Others	
compared (to/with)	MiR-34a expression in BMC was strongly upregulated in different cardiac disease patients **compared to** healthy control depicting the resemblance of cardiovascular complications with ageing.
(be)different (from) (be) dissimilar to	Because the program provides 8 hours of structured therapies daily, it **is** also **dissimilar to** both inpatient and general outpatient care.
differ (from)	Our findings **differ from** a recent study using the same data, which reported a nearly 50% relative increase in ED opioid prescribing from 2001—2010.
(be) unlike	**Unlike** the well-characterized yeast vacuole, our appreciation and understanding of the role of the lysosome in nutrient storage in mammals is only beginning to take shape.

(6) Use contrast signal words in Table 5.4 to connect the following items.

① _____ previous reports, H2 haplotype was not significantly associated with lowering of age at onset or familial FTD cases.

② These two categories did not _____ in telomere variance (difference 0.055 plus and minus 0.095, $p = 0.56$), corroborating earlier analyses.

③ In patients with clinically isolated syndrome (CIS), lower T2 intensity in the caudate nucleus was found _____ healthy controls.

④ The concentration of molecules within the droplets is adjusted such that most droplets contain no mutant genomes, _____ a small fraction contains only one.

⑤ When someone makes a choice, _____ , there is no place for indifference.

⑥ ROS have important biological properties and activities: on one hand, they serve as signaling molecules in regulatory circuits; _____ , they can damage cellular macromolecules due to their reactive nature.

⑦ _____ extensive efforts in many genetic studies, the p.A30P and p.E46K mutations have not yet been reported from any other families worldwide.

⑧ Recurrence of ENB in an extracranial ectopic site is extremely rare; _____ , this study presents 3 cases of ectopic recurrences.

(7) Use different contrast signals to write five sentences.

① _____

② _____

③ _____

④ _____

⑤ _____

(8) Writing practice

Choose one of the suggested topics and write an essay using comparison/contrast organization.

Topic suggestions:

① Precision medicine in oncology

② Translational medicine

③ Accurate immunology

④ Translational therapeutics

⑤ Clinical practice and translational medicine

2. Argumentation

Developing an argumentation or discussion is to express ideas or views, using reasons to support your opinion.

(1) Modern argumentation

The modern argumentation proposed by Toulmin (1958) consists of six building blocks: claim, grounds, backing, warrant, qualifier and rebuttals. Jenicek (2006) structured a flow chart of modern argumentation in medicine and other health sciences based on Toulmin's model of argumentation (See Figure 5.1).

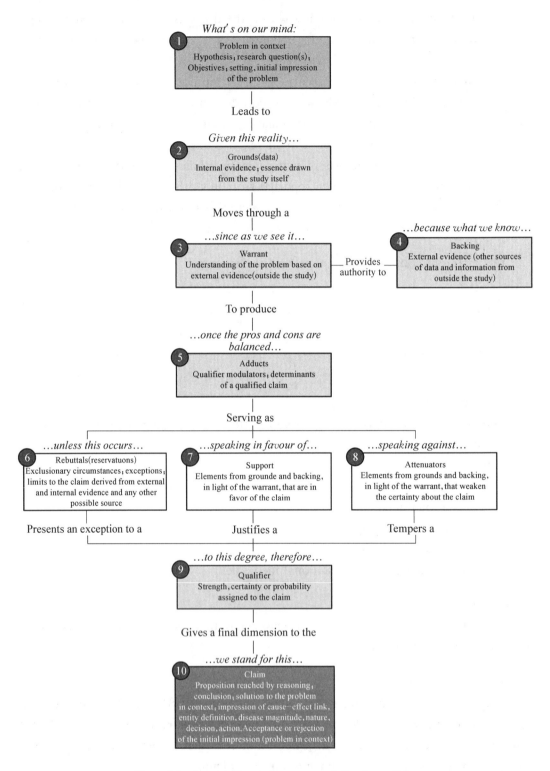

Figure 5.1 Layout of a modern argumentation in medicine

(2) Model of argumentation

The Impact of Probiotics on Male Patients
L. Paciffci et al

[1] Inflammation of the prostate or prostatitis is a very common phenomenon in adult men but also at a young age. In most cases it is not easily diagnosed considering the variable symptomatology with which it occurs, especially in cases of chronic or recurrent prostatitis (15). The triggers are often linked to lifestyle habits such as frequent travel, diets, prolonged antibiotic therapies, unbalanced nutrition, chronic constipation, psycho-physical stress, irritable bowel. Prostatitis is a disease linked to a specific cause, which must be discovered to treat the subjects in an optimal way and not to have relapses. Recognizing the cause and symptoms is very important to reduce the intensity and duration of the disease but also to avoid frequent relapses by reflecting on the patients' lifestyle habits (16).

[2] Food intolerances are extremely widespread and cause altered permeability of the intestine and consequently favor the passage of bacterial species towards the urinary tract and in particular the prostate, triggering prostatitis. Awareness of the relationship between intestinal balance and prostate well-being allows for more effective prevention and more timely treatment of prostatitis (12). Probiotics have an important role in the prevention and management of prostates but also in benign prostatic hyperplasia. This is because the "good" bacteria present in probiotics are essential for the functioning of the immune system and for the control of inflammation, key elements of both pathologies. In fact, one of the best ways to prevent prostatitis is to keep the immune system in optimal conditions. The bacteria that cause prostatitis can be controlled or eliminated by helping to improve the intestinal bacterial flora. Therefore, regular ingestion of probiotics can help prevent the development of acute and chronic prostatitis by fighting both inflammation and the possibility of infection (17).

[3] Emerging studies indicate that the microbiome can affect prostate inflammation, prostatitis/chronic pelvic pain syndrome and benign prostatic hyperplasia, as well as prostate cancer. The human microbiome present in multiple anatomical sites (urinary tract, gastrointestinal tract, oral cavity, etc.) can play essential roles such as regulation of homeostasis and the immune system and also affect systemic hormone levels (18). Recent studies seem to confirm that, in inflammatory and bone loss conditions, the use of probiotics with stem therapies could positively influence regenerative clinical practice (19 – 20).

[4] The oral microbiome is also implicated in prostate health not only for the potential to give systemic inflammation but also for the ability of some oral pathogens

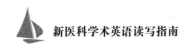
to specifically colonize the prostate. In fact, bacteria characteristic of dental plaque has been found in prostatic secretions of patients with chronic prostatitis or benign prostatic hyperplasia and, simultaneously, periodontitis (21 – 22).

[5] In a study published in 2017, 162 patients with chronic infections were recruited at various sites including 56 (35.8%) who had uro-genital inflammations to evaluate the quantitative and qualitative composition of intestinal microflora before and after treatment with probiotics. In most subjects, quantitative and qualitative changes in intestinal microflora were found, in fact, in all study groups after using probiotics, the number of pathogenic microorganisms (S.aureus, S. saprophyticus, S. epidermidis, and C.albicans) was reduced and tended to restore the normal range of the microbial landscape, inducing a reduction and improvement of the inflammatory state (23 – 24).

[6] In a study by Sherman et al., it was possible to evaluate how probiotics provide a barrier that allows the intestinal epithelium to respond to pathogenic infections (25).

[7] Resta-Lenert and Barrett have shown that probiotic bacteria are essential to protect intestinal epithelial cells in tissue culture from the adverse effects induced by the entero invasive E. coli (26 – 27). Boudeau et al. reported that a probiotic reduces both the binding and internalization of adherent and invasive E. coli strains (28). In summary, probiotic strains play an important role in attenuating host epithelial responses to pathogenic infections (29 – 39).

[8] The major limitation of our study was the small number of participants and not comparable with other probiotics and just with placebo. Another limitation of our study is not following up participants after trial completion (e.g. 3 or 6 months) to see whether their incidence of clinical and microbiological parameters changed. Further research into dosages as well as task selectivity of probiotics should be conducted in the future.

From Clin Ter 2021, 172 (1): 8 - 15

Questions for writing techniques

1. In which paragraph do the writers give background information to help readers understand the issue?
2. Does the argumentation mention initial problems? What is the research question?
3. How many grounds (internal evidence from the study itself) are given? What are they?
4. How many warrants are given? What are they?
5. How many backings are given? What are they?
6. What is the function of the last paragraph?

(3) Writing practice. Choose Topic 1 or Topic 2 and write an argumentation.

Topic 1   Agree or disagree with the following statement:

A clinician should avoid an excessive dependence on palpation and instruments.

Topic 2   Agree or disagree with the following statement:

The future status of artificial intelligence (AI) as optimal treatment and evaluating prognosis of cancers is assured.

Writing an argumentation requires careful planning.

Step 1. Revise and summarize major findings (claims) of the study.

Step 2. Succinctly remind the reader of the original thesis (statement of the problem) of the study.

Step 3. Critically appraise the evidence in grounds and its relevance to the study and its claims.

Step 4. Critically appraise both the supporting and contradictory evidence (if any) in backing and its relevance in connection to grounds and claims.

Step 5. Critically analyze and appraise the value, relevance and biological, social and technical (if any) plausibility of the warrant in general, and specifically as pertains to the study.

Step 6. Assess the link between argument building blocks and the relevance of their content to the final conclusions (claims).

Step 7. Present the final conclusions (claims) stemming from the study (or refer to Step 1), corroborating with or contradicting the original thesis as stated in Step 2 (Jenicek, 2006).

Task 3B   Moves in a medical discussion/conclusion section

The discussion section contextualizes the reported study and relates it to previous work in the field. The information can be organized as follows: (a) illustrate principal findings; (b) identify strengths and weaknesses; (c) relate strengths and weaknesses to other studies; (d) state the significance of the study; and (e) propose limitations and suggest future research. Four moves are identified in the discussion section. The first three moves are conventional, whereas the last one is optional (Kanoksilapatham, 2005; Vieira et al, 2019), see Table 5.5 and Table 5.6.

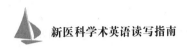
Table 5.5 Biochemistry move/step schemas for a discussion/conclusion section（Kanoksilapatham，2005）

Move 1：Contextualizing the study	Step 1：Describing established knowledge
	Step 2：Presenting generalizations，or research gaps
Move 2：Consolidating results	Step 1：Restating methodology
	Step 2：Stating selected findings
	Step 3：Referring to previous literature
	Step 4：Explaining differences in findings
	Step 5：Making overt claims or generalizations
	Step 6：Exemplifying
Move 3：Stating limitations of the present study	Step 1：Limitations about the findings
	Step 2：Limitations about the methodology
	Step 3：Limitations about the claims made
Move 4：Suggesting further research	

Table 5.6 Psychology move/step schemas for a discussion/conclusion section（Zhang et al，2011）

	Step 1：Recapitulate present research
	Step 2：Provide established knowledge of the topic
	Step 3：Highlight overall outcome
	Step 4：Compare results with previous research
	Step 5：Interpret outcome
	Step 6：Support explanation of results
	Step 7：Generalize results
	Step 8：Recommend future research
	Step 9：Indicate significance of outcome
	Step 10：Ward off counterclaim
	Step 11：Indicate limitations of outcome
	Step 12：Evaluate methodology

Task 4 Building your vocabulary

Work with your partner，match each key word and phrase to its definition.

Word/Phrase	Definition
1. consequence	**a.** declared or made legally valid.
2. capacity	**b.** the representation of what is perceived; basic component in the formation of a concept.
3. complex	**c.** the branch of medicine concerned with the birth of children.
4. highlight	**d.** the use of electronic equipment to record and display activity in the body that is not usually under your conscious control, for example your heart rate, so that you can learn to control that activity.
5. validated	**e.** complicated in structure; consisting of interconnected parts.
6. accessible	**f.** ability to perform or produce.
7. perception	**g.** serum taken from the blood of an animal and given to people to protect them from disease, poison, etc.
8. integrated	**h.** ways of resting muscular.
9. reverse	**i.** a phenomenon that follows and is caused by some previous phenomenon.
10. biofeedback	**j.** a description of how things might happen in the future.
11. serum	**k.** of words so related that one reverses the relation denoted by the other.
12. peroxide	**l.** capable of being reached.
13. prophylaxis	**m.** the branch of medicine concerned with children and their diseases.
14. algorithm	**n.** action that is taken in order to prevent disease.
15. muscular relaxation	**o.** move into the foreground to make more visible or prominent.
16. self-efficacy	**p.** true and accurate.
17. pediatrics	**q.** a clear liquid used to kill bacteria and to bleach hair.
18. scenario	**r.** formed or united into a whole.
19. authentic	**s.** the confidence whether you have the ability to produce the results that are wanted.
20. obstetrics	**t.** a set of rules that must be followed when solving a particular problem.

Task 5　Understanding the text moves

Reading 2　Text theme: Artificial intelligence in nursing

Task 5A　Read the text, and fill in each blank with a proper form of the word in the bracket.

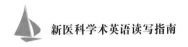

Evaluation of a Theory-Based Virtual Counseling
Application in Nursing Education
Shefaly Shorey et al

1. After incorporating certain key concepts of the social learning theory and authentic learning environment model in the development of a VP communication training program, our results revealed an improvement or maintenance of high learning attitude and self-efficacy scores among the majority of the students. Nevertheless, longitudinally, a general decline in the improvement of students' attitudes toward learning communication skills was noted. A shift in percentages from improved in self-efficacy to maintained high self-efficacy was also observed across the four scenarios. In addition, in this study, the translation of perceived self-efficacy levels into actual performance or clinical skill remains unseen, as the students were found to perform poorly in their clinical communications skill _____ (assess) compared with the previous batch, particularly in pediatrics, obstetrics, and medical settings. However, based on a follow-up qualitative study, clinical facilitators who were responsible for grading students' clinical communication skills highlighted that nonverbal communication or body language was the main areas of improvement. These objectives were not accounted for during the VP training and may have led to poorer scores among the students in the present cohort.

Learning Attitudes
2. The decline in improvement in students' learning attitudes and maintenance of low levels of positive attitudes toward communication skills could be attributed to unique challenges of using the VP simulations. In a previous study, students exposed to standardized, virtual, and traditional clinical learning environments reported that conversing with a VP was more challenging than an SP because of the limited and ____ ____ (predict) of the VP's responses. In addition, knowing that the VP was not real did not provide them with meaningful experiences. In addition, self-directed learning through VPs requires substantial self-discipline and enthusiasm as learning may wane because of a lack of face-to-face feedback from educators and peers. However, high heterogeneity between VP programs indicates the need for further qualitative analysis to examine the low and declining levels of positive learning attitudes in students.

Communication Self-efficacy
3. After the first VP scenario exposure, students' perceived self-efficacy improved significantly and remained high in the subsequent scenarios. Similarly, previous studies also reported greater increase in self-efficacy among medical students who received VP training for patient-centered interviewing and communication skills. The _____

(expose) to patients during various clinical practicums throughout the 2 years could have led to the mastery of the communication skills. According to Bandura's self-efficacy theory, four main factors enhance one's self-efficacy, which include verbal persuasion, vicarious experience, mastery experience, and the physical/emotional states of an individual. In comparison to using SPs, the use of VPs may enhance self-efficacy better as performance feedback is provided at the end of each scenario (verbal persuasion). In addition, students are able to practice together simultaneously, consult, encourage, and learn from each other during the process vicarious learning unlike with SPs. As such, students' perceived self-efficacy in clinical settings and in VP trainings could be better enhanced as compared with the use of SPs because of restricted resources.

4. Despite the decrease in the percentage of students who maintained low self-efficacy across the scenarios, the fluctuation in the number of students who improved and maintained high self-efficacy in each scenario could be due to the different scenario objectives. First, scenarios 1 and 2 were similar in terms of soliciting history-taking, rapport-building, and devising healthcare plans, which saw a higher percentage of improvement in scenario 1 and a higher percentage of maintenance in scenario 2. Scenario 3 target clinical reasoning skills and handover communication between healthcare professionals, whereby no significant improvement in self-efficacy was found. However, students in a previous qualitative study appreciated the role modeling of set handover structures (i.e., Situation, Background, assessment and Recommendations) that the VP provided. Lastly, there was a significant improvement in self-efficacy for scenario 4, which trained students to demonstrate support and empathy skills to a fellow stressed colleague. Compared with previous scenarios where students had a set interview structure, this scenario presented itself as a more personal and less structured form of communication that may have resulted in the significant improvement in the pretest and post-test scores. However, when compared with SPs, students who trained with VPs demonstrated fewer complex and nonverbal communication such as empathetic _____ (respond) and eye contact. Further research is required to examine whether the use of VPs could boost self-efficacy in providing support to others.

Clinical communication Skills

5. Although students generally had high levels of perceived communication self-efficacy after VP training, their clinical communication scores were mostly lower than the previous cohort, which did not receive VP training. This was significant for pediatric, obstetric females only, and medical males only clinical practicums. The confidence-competence gap may reflect a common issue where students overestimate the effectiveness of easy simulation training tasks. If the VP simulation was too easy,

students might believe that they have developed strong competencies from the training. Our results are in agreement with Bryant and colleagues' study, in which no significant difference was observed in course grades between students who received virtual simulations and those who did not. Because VP scenarios may be either deemed as easier or more challenging than real-life situations, VPs may not present accurate clinical scenarios, thus affecting the applicability or _____ (relevant) of the training in actual clinical settings. Based on a follow-up qualitative study, a number of recommendations such as improving speech recognition, increasing speech permutations, and having more emotional expressions and nonverbal cues could potentially enhance the authenticity of VP trainings. Furthermore, the lack of pediatric and medical VP scenarios may have contributed to the students' poor preparation for the practicums and resulted in the significant lower performance scores. In addition, the smaller sample size in the previous cohort, especially for medical practicums, could have resulted in a lower power, reduced the likelihood of a true effect, and contributed to the possibility of error inflation, thus resulting in an unfair comparison index of performance.

Limitations

6. A major study limitation was the potential bias of students' report on learning attitude and self-efficacy. Because students usually expect themselves to grow academically, this perception may influence their self-report outcomes and may not be related to the intervention implementation. Therefore, future educational interventions should adopt more valid and robust measures or a qualitative approach to investigation students' perceived benefits of a new learning program. Although the VCAAI was designed with high physical, functional, and psychological fidelity to provide optimal authenticity of the clinical settings to train communication skills, several limitations were present in the study. First, concurrent classes, assignments, and examinations led to the low sample size and high attrition. Second, the VCAAI was initially designed to be easily available and _____ (access) to students through an online platform. However, the testing of the VP simulations was unstable, and students encountered technical glitches. Hence, students were allowed only single access to the VPs at a designated computer laboratory under the supervision of laboratory technicians. The limited _____ (access) and single use of VPs may not have provided sufficient training for students to do well in their clinical communication skills. In addition, VPs were programmed in English, but as Singapore is a multicultural society, real patients often converse in their mother tongue language or dialect, thus reducing the applicability of the training to clinical settings. Lastly, the students were not randomly allocated into the intervention and control groups, thus limiting the generalizability of the finding. Given the longitudinal nature of the nursing curriculum, there could be other

confounding factors that limit the effectiveness of the intervention.

Implication for Future Research

7. Future nursing research involving the use of VPs in communication skills training should consider potential confounding variables such as demographic differences and stressors and adopt a randomized controlled trial design to provide a more accurate representation of the effectiveness of the VP simulations. Translational research is also needed to show the link between simulation and practice. A detailed outcome analysis on specific communication skill sets (eg, history-taking and handover) would also be useful to identify areas that can improve the effectiveness of future VP communication skills training. _____ (qualitatively) studies should be conduct to further evaluate the VP usage experiences of students and the conducted assessment experience of clinical facilitators. Developers should also consider including other languages and dialects to increase the authenticity of a clinical setting in a multicultural society. Furthermore, the faculty should ensure the level of complexity of the VP training is on par with a student's level of experience and develop more relevant scenarios that equip students better. Most importantly, considering that the VCAAI learning program has some limitations and scopes that it cannot cover, it should be integrated with other didactics to ensure holistic education of communication skills. Although the VCAAI was developed with nursing undergraduates in mind, its use to enhance communication skills can be adapted and applied to other healthcare education curricula as communication skills are _____ (integral) in the professional development of a healthcare provider.

From Computers, Informatics, Nursing, 2023, 41(6), 385–393

Task 5B   Read the text carefully and decide what the moves are
1. How do the authors consolidate the results?
2. How do the authors state the findings?
3. What're the main findings of this research?
4. What's the main limitation?
5. What're the suggestions for further research?

Section 2   Writing

Task 6   Warm-up writing assignment: Write an effective discussion/conclusion section

Task 6A   Grammar and phraseology in a medical discussion/conclusion section

1. Modal verbs

Modal verbs are particularly useful in a discussion/conclusion section. A possible reason，or an obvious interpretation or a probable implication should be dealt with modal verbs.

（1）Ability/capability

① Present simple：can

> Several reasons **can** be put forward to explain this lack of consensus.

② Present simple negative：cannot

> Any one of our simple categories **cannot** themselves explain the Ts-Tv fitness difference，but their combination，represented in the Ts-Tv distinction，can be quite generally predictive of fitness.

③ Past simple：could/could have

> We thus asked whether insulation by architectural proteins **could** explain some features of Hi-C contact maps that transcriptional state alone cannot.
>
> The salt sensitivity of hnRNPA1 phase behavior **could have** further led us to conclude that electrostatic interactions were key drivers of phase separation.

④ Past simple negative：could not/could not have

> Converting substrates to ABPs promoted loss-of-activity and selectivity，thus we **could not** define a single ABP capable of detecting individual apical caspases in complex mixtures.
>
> Based on parsimony，many of these losses **could not have** originated from a single common event，and instead must have occurred repeatedly and independently throughout insect evolution.

（2）Possibility/options

① Present simple：may/might/could/can

> This screen offers several advantages by increasing the number of guides testable in a single experiment to explore how diverse spacer and flanking sequences **may** affect Cas13b activity.

> High OSMR expression **might** therefore indicate a state of increased inflammatory activity among intestinal stromal cells.
>
> In particular, comparison to targets in the same family **could** be useful in understanding whether more resources should be expended on illuminating the understudied ones.

② Present simple negative: may not/might not

> Moreover, the causal relationship between population size and mode of adaptation **may not** be unidirectional.
>
> Both patterns of reproductive character displacement are highly suggestive of reinforcement and indicate that reinforcement of PMPZ barriers **might not** be a rare instance even in animals with internal fertilization.

③ Past simple: may have/might have/could have (but not can have)

> Alignment-free ONF methods however do not require a specific gene to make a prediction, and for this reason **may have** an advantage over homology-based methods.
>
> Therefore, female mice **might have** higher sensitivity to changes in eNAMPT and/or NAD + levels, and ANKI mice could provide a valuable model to address this question.
>
> The reasons for these differences are unknown, but it is feasible to speculate that cell-matrix interactions **could have** an important role.

④ Past simple negative: may not have/might not have

> Cells undergoing ferroptosis have been reported to possess only 10% of the normal levels of intracellular GSH, thus these cells **may not have** the capacity to activate caspases.
>
> These results suggest that point estimates from the bi-directional approach favor the correct model but **might not have** adequate power required for significance.

(3) Probability/belief/expectation

① Present simple：should/ought to

> Therefore，future analyses and studies **should** more deeply investigate the influence of gender in these processes.
>
> Striving for epistemic humility does not mean that clinicians **ought to** trust all patients at all times，or acquiesce to requests for medically non-beneficial interventions.

② Present simple negative：should not/ought not to

> Repetitive sequence RNAs **should not** exist alone，otherwise they interfere network formation.

③ Past simple：should have/ought to have

> The normalized coverage values were then multiplied by a factor of 2，so that genome regions with a normal diploid copy number **should have** an expected normalized coverage of 2.
>
> Finally，he argues that the happy man ought to live pleasantly. That is，if friends are pleasant to us，and if we ought to live the good life，then it ought to be pleasant to us，and therefore we **ought to have** friends.

④ Past simple negative：should not have/ought not to have

> However，given the large sample size，this limitation **should not have** a significant effect on the quantitative findings of this study，and leverage and influence analyses did not demonstrate a concerning impact of estimated variables groups on the overall study results.
>
> I take it that to call an act wrong is to say that it **ought not to** be done. If I were to say that you **ought not to have** stolen that money，then what I mean is that you **should not have** stolen that money，and that anyone in similar circumstances **should not** steal money. If someone calls an act wrong，then，it means that she believes she **should not** （and will not）do the act，nor should anyone in similar circumstances.

（4）Virtual certainty

① Present simple：must/have to

> With only a single example，this result **must** be interpreted with caution，as other causes of BRCA1/BRCA2 deficiency in this sample cannot be excluded.
>
> These findings **have to** be taken with care because force curves performed at 0.1 μm/s and 50 μm/s are both near to the experimental limits of the instrument used.

② Present simple negative：cannot

> As a predictive tool，utilizing these multiple pathogenomic mutational signatures is extraordinarily effective，with performance metrics suggesting that this method **cannot** be easily bettered.

③ Past simple：must have

> Ye et al. (2017) determined that the ancestral allele **must have** been selected in the ancestors of present-day Europeans，but located this selection in Europe，after the out of Africa bottleneck.

④ Past simple negative：cannot have/could not/could not have

> But although we **cannot have** absolute certainty in our absence calls，the phylogenetic signal in our results allows reasonable confidence that the genes we define as "missing" have truly been lost in the taxa in question.
>
> This patient was thus the exception where genetic BRCA2 nullness **could not** be proven in the tumor.
>
> Our study establishes protein degradation as a powerful approach to dissect gene regulatory factors at an unprecedented kinetic resolution that **could not have** been achieved by conventional genetic perturbation strategies.

(5) Advice/opinion

① Present simple：should/ought to

Contact for Reagent and Resource Sharing Requests for further information or reagents **should** be directed to the Lead Contact，Victor Corces（replaced-email）.

For example，we previously found that anti-PD-L1 was not effective in promoting tumor regression in the B16 melanoma model9，suggesting that additional pathways **ought to** be studied to achieve optimal tumor immunity.

② Present simple negative：should not/ought not to

When the PSV is unreliable or uninformative，we assume that the PSV **should not** be used to differentiate between the two locations and hence use a constant term（1）in the above equation.

③ Past simple：should have/ought to have

The ACS believes cancer clinical trials are vital to inform medical decisions and improve cancer care，and all patients **should have** the opportunity to participate.

④ Past simple negative：should not have/ought not have

However，because our primary aim was to compare ischaemic stroke and intracerebral haemorrhage，for which the number and timing of premorbid measurements were very similar，this study limitation **should not have** introduced any bias.

The expression would more accurately resemble，I **ought not have** disapproved of that action，and at a deeper level would be something similar to I disapprove of speaking insincerely.

(6) Necessity/obligation

① Present simple：must/need to/have to

In order to propagate，viral proteins **must** adapt to bat temperature extremes.

This potential will **need to** be further investigated and compared with existing methods for direct DNA modification detection using ONT (20, 53) or PacBio (54) sequencing.

For large organs, subsampling will need to be performed, and if paraffin processing is planned, special sampling designs **have to** be used to deal with shrinkage of subsamples during paraffin processing.

② Present simple negative: need not/do not need to/do not have to

The second criterion means that the source of the contaminant reads **need not** be present in the analyzed data set to infer contamination.

Differences in the number of parameters **do not need to** be taken into account separately, because accurate marginal-likelihood estimators naturally penalize excessive parameterization.

One immediate implication of our results is that counter to prevailing wisdom, antibody cocktails **do not have to** target distinct regions of the RBD in order to resist viral escape.

Health care professionals **do not have to** calculate risks by hand, preferable the formula should be integrated in the electronic patients records or be available in a smartphone application.

③ Past simple: needed to/had to

Further study is **needed to** understand whether choice of anesthetic technique has an influence on cognitive function after surgery during infancy.

All patients included in the study **had to** fulfill the UK Brain Bank criteria for a diagnosis of PD and were recruited from movement disorders clinics at two local National Health Service trusts.

④ Past simple negative: did not need to/did not have to/need not have

One participant, Roger, reported that he had other supports in place, and, as a result, **did not need to** access counseling.

However, we **did not have to** perform multivariate regression analyses because the imbalanced variables were not related to the outcome.

2. Modal verbs exercise

（1）Complete the sentences using modal verbs with the help of requirements in brackets

① The corresponding template molecules _____ only be characterized through the additional steps of gel electrophoresis or sequencing. (Ability/Capability)

② Restricting the possible hosts used in ONF analysis to those that are found in the respective habitat of the query virus _____ potentially increase the accuracy of prediction. (Capability)

③ This conclusion _____ be influenced by the imprecise TAD boundary calls obtained using low-resolution Hi-C data. (Possibility/Options)

④ The use of 5-mers rather than longer kmers _____ miss some more extended motifs that might cluster differently. (Possibility/Options)

⑤ Future research _____ utilise an official definition of sedentary behaviour，clearly disentangle the relationships between each biomarker and sedentary behaviour and physical activity and use objective or at the least use standardised self-report measures for assessing sedentary time. (Probability/Belief/Expectation)

⑥ The patient's lived experience _____ be in an epistemic equilibrium with the specialized clinical expertise of the clinician. (Expectation)

⑦ Our results imply that caution _____ be taken when extrapolating GWAS results from one population to predict disease risks in another population. (Virtual Certainty)

⑧ Clinical studies _____ be performed to better assess the efficacy and safety of PD-L1 t-haNK cells. (Virtual Certainty)

⑨ For a mediation to occur，there _____ been a significant indirect effect，20 meaning the effect of the independent variable through the mediatoron the dependent variable must be significant. (Virtual Certainty)

⑩ Similarly，speculation on the potential phenotypes subject to balancing selection at WFS1 _____ also be interpreted cautiously. (Advice/Opinion)

⑪ These findings suggest that Fascin level or activity _____ be tightly regulated in the nurse cells. (Necessity/Obligation)

⑫ To be included，patients _____ have undergone extensive neuropsychiatric evaluation by an experienced geriatric psychiatrist as well as a neurologist in enhanced collaboration. (Necessity)

3. Phraseology in a medical discussion/conclusion section

（1）Background information：reference to literature or research aim/question

Several reports have shown that genotypes 1 and 4 are less likely to achieve SVR compared with HCV genotypes 2 and 3.

This is consistent with several **prior studies** suggesting that these biomarkers should be combined with an ADP to achieve sufficient sensitivity for 30-day adverse events.

The main **objective of the project** is to determine a comprehensive set of factors associated with the risk for poor post-TKR outcomes in terms of severe acute or chronic persistent...

In the present study, **it was hypothesised that** regular rehabilitation including a physical exercise intervention reinforced with the addition of...

The present study was designed to investigate the frequency of stuttered speech that occurred prior to a phonetically complex word, in accordance with the first prediction of the EXPLAN model.

In the present analysis, **it was found that** the hospital in which people with stroke received their rehabilitation care contributed significantly to the variance in length of rehabilitation hospital stay.

To date, studies on aging and longevity have in general shown few consistent results and many **inconsistent results**.

(2) Statements of result: usually with reference to results section

An **interesting finding is** the safety analysis when using AAD.

The **current study found that** both the de novo PD as well as off-medicated moderate PD groups had increased functional connectivity between the more affected STN and M1S1 compared with matched control subject.

Myopic macular degeneration has been **found to cause** 12.2% of vision impairment in Japan (approximately 200 000 people).

These results **indicate** that loss of NCX3 function does not result in an upregulation of the related family member, NCX1.

The second **major finding** is that a pharmacological AC5 inhibitor, Vidarabine, replicates the salutary effects of AC5 disruption.

(3) Unexpected outcome

Surprisingly, we found widespread sIBM-specific changes in the RNA metabolism pathways themselves.

Although the direction **was unexpected**, findings are not surprising, as it may be more difficult for families with vulnerabilities in cohesion to implement...

An **unexpected finding** from our studies was the different mechanisms of growth suppression seen upon short-term (24—72 hr) versus long-term (1—2 weeks) ERK inhibitor treatment.

This finding is not **surprising** since 47% of providers noted they work in an institution that accommodates aging physicians through a change in distribution of shifts.

A **surprising** finding was that by the last follow-up most patients had a decrease of serum and CSF titers regardless of outcome.

(4) Reference to previous research: support

To determine whether these changes were **associated with** altered collagen content, we undertook circular polarization microscopic imaging of the aortic wall of 15-month-old mice.

Clinical outcomes therefore **reflect** a standardized radiation dose for all eyes involved.

These studies provide **further support** for the safety of ketamine.

Our data **confirm the association between** the two measures, with anr2correlation coefficient of 0.66, as well the finding that in patients receiving fibrinogen concentrate supplementation the level of association decreases.

This is **consistent with data obtained** in Mexico City, where 76.6% of the women included in the study viewed the medical abortion process as easy or very easy and...

Good calibration means that model-based predicted event rates closely **match those observed** in practice.

The results of our quantitative MR imaging study are **in line with those of previous studies** in which weighted signal intensity values were used for analysis of selected ROIs.

These levels and accumulation rates are **in agreement with** previously published results (Meissner et al., 2008).

In accord with the extant epidemiologic literature, covariates were considered for inclusion in the statistical models based on their meeting both of the following criteria...

(5) Reference to previous research: contradict

Although the TGFβ pathway is induced in ADO2 muscle, we were **unable to demonstrate** changes in pSmad2/3 compared to WT muscle.

Our study also identified a number of genes **not previously** implicated in antitumor immunity or resistance to immunotherapy.

Our findings are **contrary to** a recent report that lactic acid bacteria have no effect on P. larvae at the colony level.

This is **contrary to** the findings in a study in which the time interval between treatment and necropsy was 8 weeks.

We found an association between the variables diabetes and osteonecrosis, as the diabetes group had a frequency and proportion of osteonecrosis that was significantly **higher compared to** the other groups analyzed.

Although current evidence does **not support** stopping ACEI/ARB use before thoracic surgery, preoperative discontinuation of these medications may be reasonable to protect kidney function.

Although the median ISS for our study was **lower than** that of previous studies claiming a mortality benefit, ISS inflation appears to be a real phenomenon and may confound studies that use ISS to control for morbidity.

(6) Explanations for results

A **possible explanation for** this result is that more genes are involved in embryogenesis than in other developmental stages, which seems to be the case from multispecies analyses of gene expression.

This may **be explained by the fact** that MMSE and MoCA contain many test items that are insensitive to those cognitive functions that are compromised in cerebellar patients.

This may **partly be explained by** the relatively recent description of the clinical syndrome.

Some factors **could explain** these results: (a) the level of charges could play a role in the bacterial adhesion, as dentine presented lower negative charges which could reduce...

Two pathways **could explain** our observed phenotype of HO inhibition following loss of mesenchymal-derived VEGFA...

（7）Advising cautious interpretation

There is also more **uncertainty** about the integrity of the binocular system and its ability to recover after treatment in younger patients.

Next，estimates of model selection **uncertainty** were refined by bootstrapping that average fit's residuals.

Additionally，functional annotation is **somewhat limited by** only using databases with well-curated gene families，which precludes the annotation of newly characterized gene families not yet in gold standard databases.

Therefore，potentially real effects on individual traits **cannot be ruled out**.

However，our findings **cannot be extrapolated** to other organs or vascular beds.

Our results should therefore **be interpreted with caution**，in that they provide a general idea of the predicted gene family profiles based on bacteria that were functional characterized in previous studies.

It could be argued that the uptake of the released，ferritin-containing exosomes by neighboring cells diminishes the overall decrease in intracellular iron.

（8）Commenting on findings

It proved to be **rather disappointing** for controlling inflammation in other types of noninfectious uveitis.

Although the sample size is limited and measurements are from a single center，this study has **very encouraging** results.

The third major finding of our work was the **successful** translation of the CMEP in vivo.

These associations remained **significant in** multivariate models.

However，the results of this study provide **valuable** information for patients with MD and UI who are contemplating surgery.

This observation was particularly **troubling** as it has been previously reported，using similar genetic constructs，that cwn-2/Wnt is expressed at high levels in pharynx and SMD neurons in adult worms.

This finding is **reassuring** that reducing the illumination intensity will not compromise accurate detection and measurement of definitely decreased autofluorescence.

These observations are **somewhat** surprising because accumulation of muscle lactate is usually related to depletion of ATP and PCr.

（9）Suggesting general hypotheses

In sum，**these findings suggest that** Pol II drives chromatin folding such as P-P and E-P stripes at the gene level but has little or no effect on higher-order chromatin organization.

Therefore，**it is possible** that SLC25A1 activity in CSCs also relies upon IDH1 activity.

While it could **be suggested that** an archival sample was not representative of the current tumor microenvironment，it is interesting that despite this，there was still predictive value found in...

It seems that bone marrow cells can increase adiposity in response to the inhibitory LPL peptide injection.

Therefore，**it is possible** to observe a smaller stimulus-induced response magnitude in the right auditory cortex，when such a difference might not be present with a quiet background.

Therefore，**it is likely** that alterations in hippocampal structure/function，such as the ones induced by 2VO-surgery，lead to changes in pain perception.

This finding **raises the possibility** that either weekly paclitaxel or bevacizumab might be sufficient to achieve a progression-free survival benefit in patients with advanced-stage disease.

Our results **support the hypothesis** that Kv1.1 containing channels are needed to ensure accurate binaural integration in the auditory brainstem.

（10）Noting implications

Therefore，it should not **be assumed** that an ADP identifying these patients as low-risk will result in equivalent outcomes.

The clinical **implication of** this finding is that interventions to improve early linear growth may have long-term beneficial effects on stature in children born prematurely.

These results **further indicate** that tumor cell-intrinsic β-catenin activation can result in resistance to antigen-specific effector/memory T cells.

This finding has **important implications** for future trial design.

Racial disparities in CRC survival largely **reflect differences in** treatment，socioeconomic status，and comorbid-ities.

Our newly developed tissue-specific conditional Cav-1 −/− mice should **help us to** answer this question in future studies.

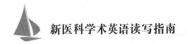
（11）Suggestions for future work

> This is an important topic for **future research**.
>
> However，there are still **unanswered questions** as to how the immune system interacts with the microbiota.
>
> A number of **questions remain** unanswered，some of which we have identified below and which can provide a basis for future research.
>
> **Future studies** will demonstrate whether drugs that prevent muscular atrophy can be used to prevent ICUAW.
>
> For this reason，**further work** is needed to enable head-to-head comparisons of antigenic evolution across these viruses.
>
> **Further research** must be performed in a lethal model to assess the value of IN IFN-I administration late in the disease course.

（12）Writing conclusions

> **To conclude**，this study has shown that the Dutch version of the OASES-S appears to be a reliable and valid instrument for providing a comprehensive assessment of the impact of stuttering in school-age children who stutter.
>
> **This study has** reviewed TARN data of 20 years of operative management of ASDH in England and Wales from 1994 to 2013.
>
> Interestingly，**this study has** also reported a decreased hazard of EDSS step 6 among patients who received immunomodulatory therapy during the progressive stage of disease.
>
> **This study has identified** clinically unrecognized variation in cognitive and gait performance in middle age associated with potentially preventable covert cerebrovascular disease...
>
> **The research has shown** that when faced with a stressor, parents apply a plethora of strategies to cope with it.
>
> **These experiments** identified 57 compounds（including mianserin）as secondary hits that produced a statistically significant increase in C. elegans lifespan.
>
> A preliminary analysis revealed that **the results of this investigation** were not affected by the menstrual cycle and thus，all participants were treated as a single group.

The results of this study indicate the presence of significant overlap of shared biological processes disrupted by large rare CNVs in children with these 2 neurodevelopmental conditions.

The resulting data can provide insights about underlying mechanisms in normal speech production.

This study **has provided** the first empirical evidence that the fetal (placental) and the maternal (blood cell) genomes harbor a lot of DNA methylation differences.

The principal **limitation of this study** is that it is retrospective in nature.

The generalizability of **this study was limited** by the fact that no women without an epidural were assigned randomly.

This study was limited to a specific community-based physiotherapy service due to the researchers' beliefs that more impact could be made on a service in which both researcher and...

The **strength of the present study** was the large number of patients having both adjustable and conventional surgery from a national database.

More research is needed to understand the complex array of factors that influence access and use of psychosocial treatments for children, and to identify strategies for improving access.

The clinical **implication** of this finding is that interventions to improve early linear growth may have long-term beneficial effects on stature in children born prematurely.

These results have significant **implications** for adult cancer survivors who face the CV effects of aging compounded by the potential detrimental impact of cancer therapy.

Task 6B   Literacy skills: Citation, references and quotations

1. The reasons/functions for citation

(1) The reasons for citation:

　① Give credit to a writer's work, acknowledge others' work;

　② Direct readers to original sources of information;

　③ Provide evidence for the writers' claims;

　④ Distinguish a writer's ideas from others;

　⑤ Avoid being accused of plagiarism.

(2) Functions of citation

According to Z. Bahadoran et al. (2020), functions of the citation in different sections of a research article are shown in Table 5.7.

Table 5.7　Functions of the citation and references in different sections of a research article

Section/Details	Functions
Introduction	Refine the research question (at least 5—10 references)
	Provide sufficient background about the study question
	Show current knowledge relevant to the study question
	Show how the study question has been previously studied
	Present concepts and variables associated with the research question
Material and methods	Elaborate the research method (at least 5—15 references)
	Describe new or previously published methods, protocols, or standards
	Describe complex or less-known statistical analyses
	Define diagnostic criteria used in the study
	Rationalize sample size estimation
	Justify specific research design or methods
Results	No reference
Discussion	Support interpretations of outcomes and conclusions (10—20 references)
	Compare the study findings with the others
	Reflect current view of the question/problem (conflicting, consensus or controversial opinions)
	Support possible explanations and implications
	Contextualize the study findings

(3) Components of the citation

The citation has three components: (1) quotation, i.e., providing either a summary, an indirect quotation (paraphrase) or a direct quotation from others' works in your own words, (2) in-text documentations, i.e., brief addressing to the source based on Harvard system or Vancouver system, etc, and (3) bibliographic details, i.e., names of authors, source of publishing, date of publishing (Bahadoran et al, 2020).

2. A quotation/reference

A quotation/reference is an acknowledgement that you are making use of other authors' arguments or data in your writing. Quotations and references are often included in NEMP research papers. They are used to support the author's ideas, voices, and findings, and sometimes to present examples or evidence. Direct and indirect quotations from reliable and knowledgeable sources are good supporting details. Direct quotation is to copy the exact words of the author, and enclose them in quotation marks. The indirect quotation is to review what the writer said in your own words. It is sometimes called reported speech (Bailey, 2003; Jordan, 2003).

E.g. Digitally enhanced monitoring is becoming an ever more important aspect of nursing practice. New surveillance technologies are applied in different contexts of nursing care, from intensive care units (Shah, 2020) to psychiatric wards (Barrera et al., 2020) and long-term care facilities (Dugstad et al., 2019) to ambient assistive living (AAL) at home (Sapci & Sapci, 2019)...

References

Barrera, A., Gee, C., Wood, A., Gibson, O., Bayley, D., & Geddes, J. (2020). Introducing artificial intelligence in acute psychiatric inpatient care: Qualitative study of its use to conduct nursing observations. Evidence-Based Mental Health.

Dugstad, Eide, Nilsen, & Eide. (2019). Towards successful digital transformation through co-creation: A longitudinal study of a four-year implementation of digital monitoring technology in residential care for persons with dementia. 19(1), 366.

Sapci, A. H., & Sapci, H. A. Innovative assisted living tools, remote monitoring technologies, artificial intelligence-driven solutions, and robotic systems for aging societies: Systematic review. JMIR Aging, 2(2), e15429.

Writing technique questions
 (1) What is the topic sentence of the paragraph?
 (2) How many reasons are there for giving references? What are they?
 (3) Mark the places where the errors occur and then write a description of the error and what is needed to correct it.

3. Discuss with your partner, identify which ones need quotations/references.
 (1) A mention of facts, data, tables or figures from another author.
 (2) An argument of your own.
 (3) Some data, tables or figures you have collected from your own research.
 (4) A theory proposed by another researcher.
 (5) A quotation from a work by any author.
 (6) Something that is consistent with common knowledge.

4. Report verbs: Use both the present and the past tenses.
It is probably best to use the present tense for recent sources or when you feel that the ideas or data are still valid. Read the following paragraph.

Recent research with newly graduated nurses **shows** how insecurity in decision-making leads to the need for a second opinion in the first place, which generally **responds to** an informal source of information, possibly based on clinical nursing practice but not always on evidence (García-Martín et al., 2021). Clinical nursing practice and clinical simulation **allow** nursing students to acquire the skills required for professional practice while also supporting them in making independent clinical decisions and cultivating social problemsolving abilities (Ahmady & Shahbazi, 2020; Gandhi et al., 2021). In this context, the effective and inclusive use of new technologies **could support** nurses and nursing students in increasing evidence-based care and decreasing low-quality services (Braithwaite et al., 2020; Hospodková et al., 2021; Saini et al., 2017), including harmful care to patients, which is estimated to account for 10% of all iatrogenic harms or adverse effects of care worldwide (National Academies of Sciences, Engineering, and Medicine et al., 2018).

From J Nurs Manag. 2022, 30:3874 – 3884, by Rodriguez-arrastia, et al

The past tense suggests that the source is older and the ideas perhaps out of date:

The preliminary content for the chatbot **was developed** by the authors based on the Reason's Swiss cheese model for patient safety (Seshia et al., 2018).

Data analysis was based on thematic analysis and supported the ATLAS.ti v9.0 software (Braun & Clarke, 2006).

5. Two main systems of reference in medical academic writing

Although many of the major journals in the medical field have adopted the Vancouver style, some still prefer the Harvard system in which the author's name and the year of publication are cited in the text.

(1) The Vancouver system, also called the numerical system

Numbers in brackets are inserted in the text for each source in the order in which they appear, and at the end of the chapter or article, the references are listed in number order. The order of the numerical system in journal articles (books) is: Author(s). Title of the paper/work. Publisher. Year of publishing. Volume. Page range. (Place of Publishing. Publisher name. Year of publishing. Number of pages P.)

E. g. A range of evidence-based treatments for depression exist, including pharmacotherapy, psychological therapies, and neurostimulation. These treatments work on average, but not all patients benefit. In fact, clinical trial data suggests that only 50% of patients respond to the initial treatment they receive, with just 30% achieving remission [1, 2]. Many patients must try multiple, sequential and/or parallel treatments on a trial-and-error basis, each taking weeks or months for potential therapeutic effects to unfold, without guarantee of success [3, 4]. This leads to sustained human suffering, accumulation of side-effects, and substantial economic costs [5, 6].

(2) The Harvard system, also called the author-and-date system

The reference is arranged by alphabetic order of the author's family name. The order of the author-date system in journal articles (books) is: Author(s). Year of publishing. Title of the paper/work. Publisher. Volume. Page range. (Place of Publishing: Publisher name. Number of pages P.) (APA, 2020)

> E.g. The rapid progress in digital innovation in health has led to a vast quantity of public and commercial digital healthcare solutions, with variable range of quality (Aryana & Brewster, 2020; Higgins, Charup et al., 2022; Marshall et al., 2020). E-mental health largely refers to the use of internet and related technologies, including phone apps, social media, or websites to offer a mental health service (Lal, 2019). Fundamental to designing optimal e-mental health innovation is a consideration of the human-computer interaction required for successful implementation (Sogaard Neilsen & Wilson, 2019).

(3) Writing practice

Write a short paragraph that develops one of the two topics given as follows. Use quotations for support. You may use them either as Vancouver system or Harvard system. Include some additional supporting sentences and transition signals to connect the ideas and make your paragraph flow smoothly.

Topic 1　Effective communication skills are the key to strengthening and enriching patient care.

_____
_____
_____
_____
_____

Topic 2　Nursing is a multifaceted profession signifying the complex task of uniting many different aspects of patient care.

_____
_____
_____
_____
_____

Tips for writing:

(a) Choose one of the topic sentences as it is given.

(b) Write several supporting sentences, using reporting verbs, main points and quotations supplied, and the techniques and rules you have learned for quotations/references.

（c）Add an in-text citation in Vancouver system or Harvard system after indirect quotation.

（d）Place the reference list at the end of the last paragraph.

（e）Use family name and initials of the given name.

Task 7　Writing task：Build a model

Task 7A　Common models and vocabulary in a medical discussion/conclusion section

1. Discuss the following questions with your partners

（1）The last sections of a medical research paper may include one of these ways. What else do you know?

Results and Discussion（combined）

Results and Discussion（separate）

Results and Conclusions（separate）

Results，Discussion and Summary（all separate）

Summary and Conclusions（separate）

（2）What is the relationship between results and discussion sections?

（3）What is the structure of a discussion/conclusion sections?

Swalesians（2012）consolidated the following findings，see Table 5.8.

Table 5.8　The Structure of a discussion/conclusion section in a research article

Move	Findings	Option/Field
Move 1	background information （research purposes，theory，methodology）	optional
Move 2	summarizing and reporting key results	obligatory
Move 3	commenting on the key results	obligatory
	（making claims，explaining the results，comparing the new work with the previous studies，offering alternative explanations）	
Move 4	stating the limitations of the study	optional
Move 5	malting recommendations for future implementation and/or for future research	optional

2. Common models of writing a medical discussion/conclusion section

The final section of the AIMRD（Abstract，Introduction，Material and methods，Results and Discussion）format used in medical research articles is discussion/ conclusion where the data found in the previous section is analyzed and discussed，see

Table 5.9.

Table 5.9　Outline of moves in medical research articles (Nwogu, 1997)

Discussion	Move 1: Highlighting overall research outcome: Confirm or refute the attainment of the main research objective	1. Using explicit preparatory statements
		2. Using explicit lexemes
	Move 2: Explaining specific research outcomes	1. Stating a specific outcome
		2. Interpreting the outcome
		3. Indicating significance of the outcome
		4. Contrasting present and previous outcomes
		5. Indicating limitations of outcomes
	Move 3: Stating research conclusions	1. Indicating research implications
		2. Promoting further research

Move 1　Highlighting overall research outcome

1. Using explicit preparatory statements

The results suggest that phonological development may hold potential for subtyping that can be explored with specific probes of phonological competency, especially at the very early stage of stuttering, a conclusion also arrived at in our earlier studies.

Our results offer insights for the development of culture systems that can improve oocyte developmental competence in vitro.

Collectively, this **study offers** evidence for the first time that commonly consumed non-antibiotic pharmaceuticals significantly promote the bacterial transformation of exogenous ARGs.

2. Using explicit lexemes

Building from our previous results, **the aim** of this study **was to determine** whether this mitochondrial dysfunction effectively impairs skeletal muscle energetics in vivo in aged rats.

The aim of the study **was to evaluate** CEUS findings in pathologically proven complicated cholecystitis (gangrenous, perforated gallbladder, pericholecystic abscess)

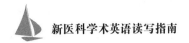
Move 2　Explaining specific research outcomes

1. Stating a specific outcome

Our results **indicated** that patients with KOA had statistically significant smaller normalized volumes of bilateral caudate nucleus and a trend toward smaller volume in the hippocampus as compared to the control subjects.

A survey of the current literature **indicated** that many of the upregulated genes have been linked to cancer and metas-tases.

2. Interpreting the outcome

This unusual result **implies that** close relatives would be disproportionally less phenotypically similar than distant relatives.

This is **particularly important** for comparison with data from experimental studies that do not collect urine samples at uniform intervals.

3. Indicating significance of the outcome

This may be **particularly important** because effective SMN-targeted therapy trials indicate a clear relationship between treatment response and timing of delivery.

4. Contrasting present and previous outcomes

Therefore，**our results indicate** that binding of proteins to clay minerals was external and provides a molecular method to observe the interaction of clay minerals-enzyme complex.

Taken together，**our results indicate** that both iron restriction and supplementation modestly attenuate colitis development in the Il10 $-/-$ colitis model.

5. Indicating limitations of the outcome

Our study included 531 individuals，representing a sub-cohort who participated in a follow-up study from the METSIM cohort（total cohort $n = 10,000$）.

Therefore，**we do not know** the time kinetics and stability of the pathway alterations revealed 6 months after behavioral testing.

Move 3   Stating research conclusions

1. Indicating research implications

> Findings from this study have important **practical implications**: First, CSF antibody determination should be included in the initial diagnostic testing; examining only serum is not sufficient.
>
> The data from the current investigation **support the concept** that AC5 inhibition reduces cancer and by syllogistic reasoning may be responsible in part for the extended longevity in this model.

2. Promoting further research

> While we interpret the robust up-regulation of GSH by CoCl2 as a compensatory response to oxidative stress, this proposed mechanism **deserves further study**.
>
> **Further studies** are also necessary to determine if and how EVs produced by osteocytes travel along the extended dendritic processes and through the LCS to the bone surface.

3. Vocabulary in a medical discussion/conclusion section

(1) Relationship to existing research

> This is **analogous to** the risk of selecting the wrong drug with current infusion pumps.
>
> These efficacy results are **comparable to** those achieved with platinum-based chemotherapy/cetuximab in the phase III EXTREME trial.
>
> These structural findings are **compatible with** our functional ones.
>
> This model is **consistent with** the reduction of efficiency associated with GMD we observed here, because reduced gray matter integrity led to the recruitment of new areas.

(2) Achievement/contribution

> While these studies **provided compelling evidence** in support of YAP1, additional modulators are likely to be revealed.

At the same time, the current study was **dramatically** smaller than case/control samples that have shown high P-value SNP associations with diagnosis.

Taken together, these studies support the **feasibility** of the second option, which is the standard approach in cochlear implant users.

(3) Limitations/future research

Future studies will be performed to investigate if the effect reported here is due to changes in inflammation or to direct effect on the microbiota.

However, **care should be taken** in implants which do not address all aspects of the complex anatomy of the distal radius metaphysis, especially the axial curvature.

In future studies, the predicted entropic changes could be tested using thermodynamic experiments designed to detect the entropic component of DNA binding.

We strongly **recommend** this approach in future host prediction studies on metagenomic viral contigs.

(4) Applications/applicability/implementation

Our approach **can be applied to** any UMI-based scRNA-seq dataset and is freely available as part of the R package sctransform, with a direct interface to our single-cell toolkit Seurat.

The approach **has potential** utility in clinical training in which the medical professionals must learn to read medical images.

These adjustments allow the exertion of high forces in acutely painful conditions but could **eventually lead to** greater fatigue and stress of the muscle tissue.

We **implement** the same averaging in the model, which enables us to make predictions for arbitrary schedules of urine collection.

Task 7B Build models and move analysis

1. Building models

(1) Elements and writing style of the discussion/conclusion section

The writing style of the discussion/conclusion is characterized by clarity, simplicity, briefness, precision and unity.

The purpose of the discussion section is to state the meaning of the results to the reader. The following elements are suggested to be included in the discussion/conclusion section (Vieira et al, 2019; Jenicek, 2006; Hess, 2004).

① State and summarize major findings (claims) of the study.

② Appraise strengths and weaknesses of the study critically.

③ Appraise strengths and weaknesses in relation to other studies critically, discussing particularly any differences in results.

④ Explain the meaning and importance of the findings.

⑤ Assess the link between the findings to those of similar studies (claims).

⑥ Consider alternative explanations of the findings.

⑦ State the clinical relevance of the findings.

⑧ Present the final conclusions (claims) stemming from the study.

⑨ Specify and justify the degree of certainty about the final claim.

⑩ Acknowledge the study's limitations.

⑪ Make suggestions for further research.

(2) Discussion/conclusion model in medical research articles

The explanation of data provided in the results section is involved in discussion/conclusion section by discussing the data, stating limitations, and providing a conclusion (Huang, 2014), see Table 5.9.

Table 5.9　Discussion/conclusion's model for medical RA

Move 1: Discuss data	Step 1: State main findings
	Step 2: Analyze the main findings
Move 2: State the limitations	Step 1: Help stating the strengths and weaknesses of the study
Move 3: Provide conclusion	Step 1: Reiterate main findings
	Step 2: Discuss implications
	Step 3: Explain how readers could further improve on the project if they ever chose to recreate it

(3) Building models for the structured discussion/conclusion section

---

Experiences and perceptions of final-year nursing students of using a chatbot in a simulated emergency situation: A qualitative study

Miguel Rodriguez-Arrastia et al

DISCUSSION

1. This study was aimed to explore the experiences and perceptions of final-year nursing students on the acceptability and feasibility of using a chatbot for clinical decision-making and patient safety.

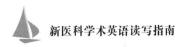
Continued

2. After analysing our results from the FGs, it was found that almost all participants reported positive feedback in terms of usability and acceptability, inferring a qualitative improvement in clinical decision-making and problem-solving abilities for patient safety in a simulated scenario. **3**. While the design and use of conversational agents for patient-chatbot interaction in niche areas such as mental health and long-term care have been widely discussed (Abd-Alrazaq et al., 2021; Fitzpatrick et al., 2017; Schachner et al., 2020), this study yields some interesting and relevant findings regarding the use of professional-chatbot interaction in order to provide precise, evidence-based and timely decisions in patient care and safety. **4**. Nursing knowledge-driven and management processes are certainly gaining traction in order to leverage the best information available to ensure the quality and safety of care provided (Braithwaite et al., 2020; Shahmoradiet al., 2017); however, to the best of our knowledge, this is the first study to explore the use of task-based AI to promote patient safety by incorporating the best evidence-based dataset into the clinical decision-making process.

5. Our findings, like those of other studies (Abd-Alrazaq et al., 2021; Dhinagaran et al., 2021), denoted that participants found the design and performance to be engaging and motivating but also improvable. **6**. Although most participant reported that the chatbot had a clean design and user-friendly navigation system, other impressions were more centred around the idea of usability and its current limitations. **7**. Suggestions included highlighting not only the most essential information or allowing users to select interface colours or colour schemes, particularly for visually impaired professionals, but also other extensions of use such as oral interaction with the conversational agent (Koman et al., 2020). **8**. Others, on the other hand, suggested that a button-based navigation system could be sufficient, if not preferred, over free-text or voice interaction, which would be especially relevant to broader accessibility and valuable for new professionals who may not know the specific information they require during their clinical decision-making process (Beilharz et al., 2021; Curran et al., 2019).

9. A number of studies are currently looking for new approaches to integrate chatbots and AI-based conversational agents to support health-related activities, albeit the quality of content still needs to be improved (Park et al., 2019; To et al., 2021). **10**. While the information was found to be adequate, accessible and useful, nearly all participants felt that the content output could be more concise, accurate and employ appropriate length responses and also include other options to motivate participants to explore other related content at their own pace (Stal et al., 2021). **11**. One possible explanation for this could be the need of different levels of chatbot personalization (intrinsic, extrinsic or a mix of both) in order to create user profiles or user models and support personalized and adaptative features (Fang et al., 2018; Kocaballi et al., 2019). **12**. Indeed, earlier research has shown that adaptative conversational approaches such as determining level of expertise or confirmation strategies can improve system performance, usability and efficacy in clinical decision-making, resulting in increased accuracy and patient safety (Abd-Alrazaq et al., 2021).

13. These technologies may support organizations, senior nurses and other health managers in reducing biassed judgement and decisionmaking at both the individual and group levels, which may have a negative impact on patient safety at all levels of the health system (Mannion & Thompson, 2014). **14**. Based on our findings, however, there are certain challenges to be considered when integrating conversational agents in real nursing practice. **15**. Whereas there appears to be a positive mindset and self-efficacy toward adopting a chatbot, adequate resources, time, training and knowledge are required to support acceptance and long-term use among nursing students and professionals (Brandtzaeg & Følstad, 2018; Følstad et al., 2018). **16**. This technology may support nurses and nursing students in making informed decisions during the patient care by automating the data process; however, the final clinical decision should rely on their clinical judgement, considering current evidence and a view of appropriate clinical practice (Akbar et al., 2021; Araujo et al., 2020). **17**. It should be noted that there may be professional concerns and reservations about using chatbots,

Continued

including fear or uncertainty for the unknown, ethical and privacy implications or the perception of additional workload (Mokmin & Ibrahim, 2021). **18**. For these reasons, recent research suggests that front-line professionals should be involved in the design and implementation of decision-making support systems, sharing their perspectives and verbalizing their perceptions and underlying nursing practice requirements, thereby promoting a better adoption of their use for care quality and patient safety (Fritz & Dermody, 2019). **19**. Despite these findings lend weight to the idea that the digital age and the speed with which information is transmitted are transforming communications and clinical practices, the research on the use of conversational agents in nursing practice for patient safety is still limited (Curran et al., 2019; Rouleau et al., 2017). **20**. This could be explained by the fact that the most current software available for implementing conversational agents is fee-based and thus not cost-effective to maintain in clinical practice (Barthelmäs et al., 2021). **21**. Surely, some participants mentioned the usefulness and beneficial effects that such advances may have in promoting evidence-based clinical decisionmaking at the bedside, regardless this technology is not currently present in their actual clinical placements (Martinez-Garcia et al., 2021). **22**. Emerging information and communication technologies, such as AI-based conversational agents, may not only contribute in better patient safety judgements and decisions but also introduce new avenues for higher organizational safety culture values (Akbar et al., 2021). **23**. The use of more transparent knowledge sharing among organizational members through use of reliable resources may improve clinical decision-making abilities of nurses and develop methods for using common knowledge at an organizational level to promote trust and organizational culture (Yoo et al., 2019).

24. Conversely, there are important limitations to consider when interpreting our results. **25**. Given the exploratory nature of our study, nursing students were chosen to avoid potential technological barriers using a homogeneous sample within an uncommon clinical situation. **26**. Nursing students were only expected to interact with the task-based chatbot using a specified individual case scenario, a pesticide poisoning patient in primary care settings. **27**. This study also lacks a concrete measure for evaluating the chatbot interaction. **28**. Although there are considerable inventories for evaluating evidence-informed decisionmaking competence in nursing practice and training interaction with chatbot (Belita et al., 2021; Mokmin & Ibrahim, 2021), no studies have been found to explore the use of a toolkit to assess nurses-chatbot conversations pertaining patient safety. **29**. To the best of our knowledge, no study has yet focused on the design of a chatbot for student or professional-chatbot interaction in clinical decision-making and patient safety, which has limited our discussion. **30**. Rather than concluding this topic, however, our findings warrant further discussion. **31**. Future research should explore a gamut of clinical scenarios and may use our preliminary findings to provide a more sophisticated chatbot design. **32**. A future challenge for the chatbot should be to include professional nurses and account for their needs in the design for accuracy, as well as to include other advanced forms of chatbots such as AI-based conversational agents with deeper levels of extrinsic personalization.

CONCLUSIONS

33. The findings of our study provide preliminary support for the acceptability and feasibility of adopting a chatbot for clinical decision-making regarding nursing care and patient safety in certain situations, although more research using diverse methodological approaches is required. **34**. Our results revealed not just an overall positive response to the design, performance and content output but also substantial recommendations for refining navigation, layout and content, as well as useful insights to support its acceptance in real nursing practice. **35**. SafeBot may constitute a down-to-earth resource to help cover gaps in service delivery in terms of patient safety and to support clinical decision-making with appealing and easily available evidence-based information.

From J Nurs Manag. 2022, 30(8): 3874–3884

2. Move analysis: Analyze the move structures

In Sentences 1 – 2, the writers present generalization of the research, and summarize overall research outcome (claims) of the study.

In Sentences 3 – 4, the writers appraise strengths and weaknesses in relation to other studies critically, discussing particularly any differences in results.

In Sentences 5 – 8, the writers interpret the outcome, and assess the link between the findings to those of similar studies (claims).

In Sentences 9 – 12, the writers interpret the outcome, and relate the findings to those of similar studies.

In Sentences 13 – 23, the writers restate the methodology, indicate significance of the outcome, and contrast present and previous outcomes.

In Sentences 24 – 29, the writers indicate limitations of outcomes.

In Sentences 30 – 32, the writers make suggestions for further research.

In Sentence 33, the writers reiterate main findings.

In Sentence 34, the writers indicate research implications.

In Sentence 35, the writers promote further research.

3. The model rebuilt

We may streamline the move analysis above to reconstruct the model for a discussion/conclusion section as follows:

Moves	Steps
Move 1: Contextualizing overall research results	Step 1: Presenting generalization of the research Step 2: Providing established knowledge of the topic Step 3: Stating the major results
Move 2: Interpreting specific research findings	Step 4: Restating methodology Step 5: Stating specific findings, and summarizing overall research outcome (claims) of the study. Step 6: Appraising strengths and weaknesses in relation to other studies critically, discussing particularly any differences in results. Step 7: Interpreting the outcome, and assessing the link between the findings to those of similar studies. Step 8: Refining significance/achievement/contribution of the outcome. Step 9: Acknowledging limitations of the outcome.
Move 3: Stating research conclusions	Step 10: Indicating research implications/applications. Step 11: Promoting further/future work

Task 8   Final assignment: Write an effective discussion/conclusion section

Search "Artificial intelligence in treatment" or "Artificial intelligence in nursing" on the internet, or use a sample provided by your instructor. Write an effective discussion/conclusion section about "Artificial intelligence in treatment" or "Artificial intelligence in nursing" using your descriptions of extended comparison and contrast.

Your discussion/conclusion should contain

- Revising previous sections
- Highlighting overall research findings
- Stating specific findings
- Interpreting the findings of the present work
- Comparing strengths and weaknesses in relation to other studies critically
- Indicating significance of the outcome
- Contrasting present and previous outcomes
- Acknowledging limitations of findings
- Indicating research implications/applications
- Promoting further/future work

Further reading

American Medical Association. AMA Manual of Style Committee. (2020). *AMA Manual of Style: A Guide for Authors and Editors*, (11th ed). New York: Oxford University Press.

American Psychological Association. (2020). *Publication manual* of the American psychological association (7th ed.).

Bahadoran, Z., Mirmiran, P., Kashfi, K., et al. (2020).The Principles of Biomedical Scientific Writing: Citation. *Int J Endocrinol Metab*, 18(2):e102622.

Bailey, S. (2003). *Academic writing: A practical guide for students*. London & New York: Routledge.

Barten, D. L. J., Pieters, B. R., Bouter, A., et al. (2023). Towards artificial intelligence-based automated treatment planning in clinical practice: A prospective study of the first clinical experiences in high-dose-rate prostate brachytherapy. *Brachytherapy*, 22(2):279 – 289.

Berridge, C., Grigorovich, A. (2022). Algorithmic harms and digital ageism in the use of surveillance technologies in nursing homes. *Front Sociol*. 7:957246.

Calabresi, P. A., Kappos, L., Giovannoni, G., et al. (2021). Measuring treatment response to advance precision medicine for multiple sclerosis. *Ann Clin Transl Neurol*. 8(11):2166 – 2173.

Carson, J. M., Barbieri, S., Matthews, G. V., et al. (2023). National trends in retreatment of HCV due to reinfection or treatment failure in Australia. *J Hepatol*, 78(2):260 –270.

Ciancarelli，I.，Morone，G.，Tozzi，M. G.，et al. (2022). Identification of Determinants of Biofeedback Treatment's Efficacy in Treating Migraine and Oxidative Stress by ARIANNA (Artificial Intelligent Assistant for Neural Network Analysis). *Healthcare (Basel)*, 10(5):941.

de Santiago，I.，Polanski，L. (2022). Data-Driven Medicine in the Diagnosis and Treatment of Infertility. *J Clin Med*, 11(21):6426.

Hess，D. R. (2004). How to write an effective discussion. *Respiratory care*, 49(10), 1238 – 1241.

Huang，D. (2014). Genre analysis of moves in medical research articles. *Stylus*, 5(1), 7 – 17.

Jenicek，M. (2006). How to read，understand，and write "Discussion" sections in medical articles. An exercise in critical thinking. *Med Sci Monit*, 12(6):SR28 –36.

Jiang，N.，Xie，H.，Lin，J.，et al. (2022). Diagnosis and Nursing Intervention of Gynecological Ovarian Endometriosis with Magnetic Resonance Imaging under Artificial Intelligence Algorithm. *Comput Intell Neurosci*, 2022(1):3123310.

Jordan，R. R. (2003). *Academic Writing Course-Study Skill in English*. Harlow：Pearson Education

Kanoksilapatham，B. (2005). Rhetorical structure of biochemistry research articles. *English for specific purposes*, 24(3), 269 – 292.

Lee，C. T.，Palacios，J.，Richards，D.，et al. (2023). The Precision in Psychiatry (PIP) study：Testing an internet-based methodology for accelerating research in treatment prediction and personalisation. *BMC Psychiatry*, 23(1):25.

Makar，G.，Foltz，C.，Lendner，M.，et al. (2018). How to Write Effective Discussion and Conclusion Sections. *Clin Spine Surg*, 31(8):345 – 346.

Oshima，A.，& Hogue，A.(2006). *Writing academic English*. Longman.

O'Connor，S. (2022). Teaching artificial intelligence to nursing and midwifery students. *Nurse Educ Pract*, 64:103451.

Pacifici，L.，Santacroce，L.，Dipalma，G.，et al. (2021). Gender medicine：the impact of probiotics on male patients. *Clin Ter*. 171(1):e8 – e15.

Ribeiro，O. M. P. L.，Coimbra，V. M. O.，Pereira，S. C. A.，et al. (2022). Impact of COVID-19 on the Environments of Professional Nursing Practice and Nurses' Job Satisfaction. *Int J Environ Res Public Health*. 19(24):16908.

Rodriguez-Arrastia，M.，Martinez-Ortigosa，A.，Ruiz-Gonzalez，C.，et al. (2022). Experiences and perceptions of final-year nursing students of using a chatbot in a simulated emergency situation：A qualitative study. *J Nurs Manag*. 30 (8)：3874 –3884.

Rubeis，G. (2023). Adiaphorisation and the digital nursing gaze：Liquid surveillance in long-term care. *Nurs Philos*. 24(1):e12388.

Sandvik, A. H., & Hilli, Y. (2023). Understanding and formation—A process of becoming a nurse. *Nursing Philosophy*, 24(1), e12387.

Shorey, S., Ang, E. N. K., Ng, E. D., et al. (2023). Evaluation of a Theory-Based Virtual Counseling Application in Nursing Education. *Comput Inform Nurs*. 41 (6): 385 – 393.

Swales, J. M., & Feak, C. B. (2012). *Academic writing for graduate students: Essential tasks and skills* (3rd). Ann Arbor, MI: University of Michigan Press.

Toulmin, S. E. (2003). *The uses of argument*. Cambridge and New York: Cambridge university press.

Vieira, R. F., Lima, R. C. D., & Mizubuti, E. S. G. (2019). How to write the discussion section of a scientific article. *Acta Scientiarum. Agronomy*, 41:e42621.

Wilson, R. L., Higgins, O., Atem, J., et al. (2023). Artificial intelligence: An eye cast towards the mental health nursing horizon. *Int J Ment Health Nurs*. 32(3): 938 – 944.

Zhang, L., Kopak, R., Freund, L., et al. (2011). Making functional units functional: The role of rhetorical structure in use of scholarly journal articles. *International Journal of Information Management*, 31(1), 21 – 29.